DID YOU KNOW . . .

Baldness isn't always hereditary.

Causes for baldness and hair loss include:

* Losing weight   * Bacterial infections
* Skin disorders   * Nutritional deficiencies
* Stress   * Hormonal imbalances

Baldness is reversible!

In BALD NO MORE, Dr. Morton Walker tells you how to identify the cause of your hair loss and explains what you can do to stop the spread of baldness and restart hair growth. Citing case studies and clinical tests performed on people suffering from hair loss, Dr. Walker explains the benefits of taking nutritional supplements and soybean products, and of using the amazing Thymu-Skin® shampoo and lotion.

No more excuses!

Discover the latest health tips and proven results and become—

BALD NO MORE

BALD NO MORE

MORTON WALKER, D.P.M.

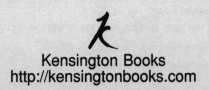

Kensington Books
http://kensingtonbooks.com

KENSINGTON BOOKS are published by

Kensington Publishing Corp.
850 Third Avenue
New York, NY 10022

Kensington and the K logo Reg. U.S. Pat. & TM Off.

First Kensington Paperback Printing: July, 1998

Printed in the United States of America
10 9 8 7 6 5 4 3 2 1

To my son, Jules Louis Walker, who at age thirty-three has the opportunity to restore lost hair growth and retain remaining hair for the rest of his life despite the potential for male pattern baldness which he probably acquired genetically or hormonally from me.

Disclaimer and Disavowal of Responsibility

This book has been written and published strictly for informational purposes, and in no way should be used as a substitute for advice from one's own health care professional.

Educational material found here should not be considered to replace consultation with a dermatologist or other medical practitioner. However, almost all the facts in this book have come from laboratory and/or clinical studies, scientific publications, consumer books, or interviews with informed health care personnel such as general physicians, oncologists, dermatologists, gynecologists, internists, medical statisticians, and other health professionals or from their patients who have experienced hair loss. Photographs included depict the actual patients participating in treatment programs.

Unless indicated otherwise as by footnotes, the identities of patients, including their occupations, residence or work locations, including their direct quotes, are fictional in this book. However, the research scientists quoted, especially the German medical doctors and professors conducting clinical studies cited, are authentic. Their statements are taken from tape-recorded interviews conducted by the author or from published or unpublished research papers that they had contributed for inclusion here.

German university medical professors and other doctors have provided scientific facts, case histories, and published or unpublished laboratory or clinical investigations. Even so, it is emphasized that none of the information imparted should be considered as the practice of medicine. The author and publisher of this book, as well as the therapeutic, nutritional, and/or cosmetic product suppliers mentioned herein, are merely providing educational material for informational purposes.

Please take the above message as a disclaimer. It's the disavowal of all responsibility by the author, publisher, and product suppliers for any practice, technique, method, knowledge or other information acted upon or taken from this book.

Contents

Foreword

Hair on the head greatly influences an individual's appearance, a phenomenon of such importance that baldness often leads to severe psychological and/or sociological disturbances. Yet, there's no single answer as to why baldness occurs because it comprises several different diseases of known pathogeneses. Various therapeutic approaches have therefore been developed to counteract baldness, and until now the rate of success of the majority of them has not been satisfactory.

In this new, updated, and greatly expanded second edition of his original book, *How to Stop Baldness and Regrow Hair,* Dr. Morton Walker provides us with much information about using diet, phytochemicals, enzymes, herbs, nutrients (including vitamins, minerals, and essential fatty acids), plus many nutraceuticals for the restoration of a healthy head of hair. He also gives details about getting to the root of your hair problem by use of scalp stimulators, massage, plus proper washing, drying, and brushing techniques for head hair. Not forgotten or discounted either are methods of hair replacement including flap surgery, hair transplants, hairpieces, and the correct stylings to camouflage thinning hair.

Yet, there is even greater knowledge to be acquired on these pages about another, more important alternative method for restoring hair growth. It's calf thymus extract—

imported to America from Mannheim, Germany. This well-developed and promising therapeutic concept has emerged during the past decade. It incorporates calf thymus extract as the viable agent of treatment for hair loss by substituting for insufficient human thymus hormone (thymosin). Located high in the chest cavity extending upwards into the neck to the lower edge of the thyroid gland and downwards as far as the fourth costal cartilage, one's thymus gland is a vital organ of the human body. Most significantly, it acts as a regulator of each person's immune system.

The thymus affects one part of the maturation of T-derived lymphocytes. These T-lymphocytic cells are one particular type of the two forms of white blood cells. They encourage secretion of thymus peptides into the blood to influence various cellular systems and are very important for human survival. The thymus gland produces such T-cells. As an individual ages, however, his or her thymus gland shrinks, and this condition correlates with augmentation of autoimmune diseases. That hormone from the thymus—thymosin—is absolutely vital for effective immune system functioning.

In Europe, the administration of total thymus extract against autoimmune diseases such as rheumatoid arthritis and systemic lupus erythematosis has a long tradition. Thymus is employed for the treatment of cancer and infectious diseases, too. Effective thymus compounds in the form of low molecular peptides now have been created for use against different types of baldness in the form of a new topically-applied product.

Local applications of *Thymu-Skin*® lotion, gel, and shampoo are providing outstanding results for the prevention of baldness in cancer patients who require chemotherapy. When massaged into the scalp right from the beginning of cytotoxic therapy, *Thymu-Skin*® prevents the cancer patient's hair from falling out. Even more remarkable is the excellent hair regrowth being experienced by patients with long-standing total baldness (alopecia areata totalis). These results are spectacular.

To explain what and how *Thymu-Skin*® accomplishes its

fine therapeutic effects, we have the second edition of this exceedingly well-written and easy-to-read book by that renown medical journalist Dr. Morton Walker. He has been well-received in Germany, Austria, and other German-speaking countries. For consumers outside of the medical field, *Bald No More: How to Stop Baldness and Regrow Hair* discusses the most important hair diseases and then demonstrates the existing results of the *Thymu-Skin®* treatment program.

While Dr. Walker's writing technique is truly admirable, at the same time it's astonishing for me to observe how professionally he achieves his task of clearly and succinctly explaining the highly complex science of hair follicle anatomy, hair growth, hair loss, and the hypotheses related to these subjects. He has an excellent way of presenting data, including hard statistical results, which normally aren't exciting to read.

Using a sophisticated network of personal experiences, patient histories, and successful treatments, Dr. Walker effectively teaches us about the scalp, hair loss, and hair regrowth. This book is a superb adviser for those suffering from almost any kind of hair loss. By broad distribution of Dr. Walker's message, many millions of balding men and women worldwide may become happy once again. I verify that this book tells the truth about how to stop baldness and regrow hair, and I'm happy to have furnished the foreword for the first edition and now the second one as well. *Bald No More: How to Stop Baldness and Regrow Hair* is the most succinct but complete popular mass market trade book ever written for comprehension by the intelligent and educated medical consumer.

> —Professor and Doctor of Medicine Manfred Hagedorn, M.D., Medical Director, Dermatology Department, Municipal Clinics of Darmstadt; Chief of the Dermatology Department at the University of Frankfurt in Damnstadt, Germany.

PREFACE

The author of a 1988 book about traveling the world's circumference at the equator Thurston Clarke, tells the discomforting story of his first exposure to personal hair loss.[1] The troubling experience happened when he was just seventeen years old.

Young Clarke employed the services of a bald barber named Antonio Sambito who usually cut the hair of Thurston's fellow classmates in the brightly lighted basement of a boys' boarding school in Massachusetts.

"I was sitting in Mr. Sambito's barber chair," writes the author, "receiving his customary five-minute bowl haircut, when he said, 'I got bad news for you, Clarke. It's going!'"

"What's going?"

"Your hair, buddy."

The barber held up a mirror so that the student could see the top of his head. A small oval patch not yet bare, but lighter in color than the surrounding territory had made its appearance. The young man reached back to touch the silky depression in his hair, and felt faint. His father had prepared him for this potential event, for Mr. Clarke senior had gone bald early in life as had his own father, and Thurston's mother's father, too.

"I knew I would finally follow them, but, my God, so soon?" wondered the young man. "I lowered my eyes to the floor—anything to avoid seeing that spot." Then, after a prolonged pause, the innocent seventeen-year-old asked, "What stops it, Mr. Sambito?" He believed this authoritarian-like barber would have the answer to pending baldness because he was an adult—wearing a white coat—who cut hair as his means of livelihood.

"Only one thing stops hair falling," the barber declared.

"What, what, Mr. Sambito? What will stop my hair from falling," pleaded Thurston, whose thinning hair did eventually disappear by the time he turned a mere twenty-five years old.

With a certain brightness reflecting off his own shining pate from sunlight streaming through the school's basement window, and a knowing smile framing his colorless lips, Antonio Sambito replied, "I used it myself, and it works every time. You know what it is, buddy? The only thing that stops hair from falling further?"

"What, Mr. Sambito, what?" Thurston Clarke again asked, on the verge of tears.

Antonio answered, "The floor!"[2]

Young Thurston Clarke was *not* amused then and he feels even more vexation now, upon recalling that long-ago incident.

The Control of Hair Growth Is Possible Today

There's been a breakthrough that addresses major hair and scalp problems affecting millions of men and women around the world. The control of hair growth is possible today.

Yes, it's true! Stopping baldness and regrowing hair that was once thought completely lost can be accomplished. The statement that one can overcome hair loss and restore its growth may have at one time seemed silly or at the least presumptuous, but now this bodily response is quite possible.

Certainly this statement would have gotten a belly-laugh

from the conservative scientific establishment thirty years ago, a snicker twenty years ago, and a raised eyebrow ten years ago. Since then, it has been understood as verifiable that someday soon, medical science would find a way to achieve man's (and woman's) age-old dream—to stop baldness and reignite one's natural hair growth process.

Now that dream has largely been realized, and controlling the hair growth process by means of diet, nutritional supplements, and the topically applied combination of products actually has happened. Researchers have made a particular externally applied compound a reality. Along with information about nutrients that nourish one's hair follicles, this new aggregate of shampoo and hair revitalizer containing calf thymus gland extract is the primary subject of my book.

Its discovery, development, production, North American importation, and sale are all predicated on the fact that the Food and Drug Administration (FDA) of the United States finally accepted in 1989 that hair growth could be positively increased by non-drug cosmetic applications directly to the scalp. Informed hair scientists in Germany, Japan, China, France, Switzerland, and the United States all began developing treatments which individually affected hair growth. For at least half-a-dozen years, they had worked diligently but independently to perfect an extrinsically-applied lotion, liniment, gel, spray, cream, or ointment to stimulate hair regrowth or to prevent the further falling of hair.

One might wonder, which scientists among the several competing nations would emerge with the master treatment? Which of the many approaches produced the best and safest results? Which therapeutic procedure could be applicable cosmetically to just about everyone?

The FDA decision had smashed the old certainties about hair and what causes it to grow or fall out. So, who now among the many countries involved could have put together the new answers on controlling hair growth? Everyone involved wondered, whose formulation would prove itself to be most valid?

In the international race to be first with a safe, viable, easily applicable, fair-priced, scalp-stimulating product that excites hair follicles into growth action, competition was keen. Each investigator knew that the rewards would be great.

Saving One's Hair by Means of German Ingenuity

German scientists were the first to perfect the means to stop baldness (alopecia) and regrow hair. Involved in the research to bring a hair stimulating product to market were some of Germany's top biologists, chemists, dermatologists, gynecologists, oncologists, internists, and entrepreneurs. What's been done for balding people worldwide is marvelous.

While populated by one of the oldest established people of Europe, the political entity of Germany today is the youngest of the European great powers. In their periods of productivity, German scientists have worked along lines pursued by those in other countries, pioneering in some fields, following in others, and often making significant contributions to the fund of world knowledge.

Ingenuity among German scientists has netted them 22.3 percent of the awarded Nobel prizes to date—second only to the United States. They have overcome the earlier decimation of Germany's scientific ranks during World War II, when many Nobel laureates were driven out of the country for political or religious reasons. These included the chemists Fritz Haber and Richard Willstater, the biochemist Otto Meyerhof, the physicist James Franck, and the physicist/mathematician, Albert Einstein.[3]

The entrepreneural genius of Guenther H. Klett-Loch who resides in Mannheim, Germany deserves special recognition. Herr Klett-Loch is responsible for combining thymus gland extract with certain herbs and other natural ingredients to create today's remedy for regrowing hair, Thymu-Skin®, to which all of us now have access. Yet, according to recorded history, hair restoration wasn't always so accessible. Investigations into stopping baldness and regrowing hair began at least sixty centuries ago.

A History of Baldness Research

Throughout the history of humankind, people have been obsessed with their hair, equating luxurious locks with youth, virility, stamina, strength, beauty, and sensuality. For as long as records have been kept, hair on the head has been considered a sexual object. For thousands of years, its texture, styling, length, color, and other attributes have been among the charismatic standards of adornment in almost every civilization.[4]

Do you know why Julius Caesar wore a wreath of leaves? It was to hide his hair loss—a receded forehead and bare-scalp crown. In some cultures, women, prisoners and soldiers are forced to hide their hair or shave it to symbolize a lack of individuality or sexuality. Look at what happens to the heads of recruits newly entered into a nation's armed forces. Their heads are clean-shaven both to take away dignity and to separate them from being distinct entities unto themselves. Removing head hair makes someone a non-person with no distinct identity.

Charles Berg, a psychoanalyst of the Freudian school, believed that the normal concern about the hair becoming thin, falling out or greyish, was a displacement of castration anxiety and that shaving the head was symbolic castration. This explanation may seem extreme, but in some societies and religions, shaving the head is associated with celibacy or chastity, as is to a lesser extent covering the hair in Muslim and orthodox Jewish society.[5]

Periods of time throughout the 1900s have been defined by certain hairstyles or haircuts such as the 1920s "spit curl," the 1950s "beehive" for females and "ducktail" for males, the 1980s "bob" for women and long hair for men, and the 1990s "mohawk" for both sexes. The importance and role of hair all through history and how it is viewed in today's society identifies ways in which people try to fit into the "mane" stream of society despite the incidence of baldness.

Hair connotes power and has symbolized sturdiness for men. When Delilah cut off Samson's hair, he lost the great strength which characterized him. So he was captured by the Philistines. In the Bible (Judges 16:17), Samson is quoted as saying: "If I be shaved, then my strength will leave me, and I shall become weak, and be like any other man."

American Indian warriors believed that when they scalped the enemy they would possess his strength and courage. The warrior with the greatest number of scalps was considered the most powerful.[6]

Documented research into hair loss and hair growth goes back 6,000 years to Egypt's Ancient Kingdom. The pharaohs had an exotic concoction of crocodile glands, owl blood, ibex fat, and mineral salts which had little basis in science, but it was a great way to reduce the crocodile, owl, and ibex populations.

The Greek philosophers furnished words of advice on growing hair; and the Roman Stoics thought that this whole subject should be ignored.

Medieval alchemists advised the use of powdered unicorn horn among other ingredients. Who knows? It might have worked if unicorns were more plentiful.

Native American medicine men found a hair-growing use for the black, smelly ooze now called petroleum—a first class hair tonic, they thought.

As late as the 1900s, X-irradiation seemed a good idea and was applied for hair restoration purposes too. One wonders what numbers of human scalps and the brain cells under them had gotten fried and shrunken from X-ray machine usage?

Emotional Depression Among the Bald

Another question arises: how many balding men and women become emotionally depressed as a result of what they believe to be an overwhelming affliction? In her book, *The Big Fall: Living with Hair Loss,* Sheila Jacobs of Vancouver, British Columbia, Canada, tells how as a result of alopecia universalis (total fallout of hair on all body parts), she permanently lost all of her hair, including the eyebrows, eyelashes, under the arms, and across the pubic region. In 1987, Ms. Jacobs wrote:

> Hair loss turns out to be more like a game of snakes and ladders than a problem with a solution. It affects self-esteem, and that affects almost every aspect of life. The only way I have found to cope with it is to remain flexible, vulnerable, and humble—willing to help others, but ready to learn and accept help too, and even ask for it.

Sheila Jacobs suffered from an emotional problem directly related to her baldness, and in her book, she explained her depressing experience and discussed how she finally was able to cope with it.[7]

In contrast, my book focuses on providing information about the nutritional feeding of hair follicles to awaken them from dormancy and the actual, topically applied, physiological solution for baldness that comes from certain pathological causes. The following introductory chapter, touches briefly on key points that will be explored in depth in full chapters.

As well as explaining the methods for achieving actual hair restoration, I will be discussing the modern human's hairy origins, and his or her hair follicles' anatomy. You'll learn about the relatively common hair and scalp disorders, and about several disturbances in body image some people experience consciously and subconsciously from their hair loss.

I'll conclude with what you really want to know: how to return hair growth to what it had been in younger years when you sported a lustrous mop atop your head.

The answers for how to stop baldness and regrow hair are available in this book. You *can* have new hair growth and you *can* keep it permanently!

Hair growth and hair styling have long been recognized in anthropological and psychiatric literature. Its associated with the concept of attractiveness, power, physical strength, and attaining goals. As opposed to how hair was considered by primitive peoples, in modern humans, it has practically no other significance than as a sexual symbol.

For anyone functioning as a psychologically normal person, it's usual for there to be a small degree of hair fetishism. However, some victims of alopecia have asserted that they would prefer to be without an arm or a leg or an eye than minus head hair. Even minimal facial hair in a glamorous woman may cause her great distress.

These various psychological effects related to the presence or absence of hair are frequently not based upon reality value. Instead, like nearly all of the effects connected with head hair, they probably have their source in profound unconscious clustering about the central idea of the importance of showing the head as a display piece. Hair on the head is like plumage for a peacock!

That's why some men with quite mild male pattern baldness (androgenetic alopecia) caused by excessive testosterone will go to great lengths to improve their appearance by prosthetic (hairpiece) and/or surgical (hair transplant) means. I did this myself thirty years ago when I invested thousands of dollars in three toupees.

Confirmation lies around us everywhere. Hair is important as a component of the body image. Many of us feel compelled to stop our baldness and start regrowing hair.

I have written this book to reeducate those adult men and women who have lost their hair and lost any hope of regaining it. The same situation once described me, but during a research trip to Germany in October 1994 I came upon a remedy for my own male pattern baldness. From being bald as a cue ball, I am again growing hair strands where there had been none for over thirty years. While there hardly are enough of them, some of these new hairs are three inches long and they continue to grow longer.

There is much to know about restoring hair growth on the head, so let's begin the learning process.

—Morton Walker, D.P.M.
Stamford, Connecticut
December 31, 1997

INTRODUCTION

Right up front, I am compelled to disclose that some have questioned my credentials as a hair folliclely-wise man of the moment. It's true that I do fit in quite well with those forty-four million or more American men who show bald heads or who exhibit definite signs that their hair is on the way out. Across my forehead and crown much more skin than hair makes its appearance. I am bald, a condition quite apparent to observers for about forty years.

Comedian Jay Leno, host of WNBC's "The Tonight Show with Jay Leno," held up the smaller first edition of this book, and milked a good laugh from the back cover picture of its author—me—with my mostly bare head showing.

I'm sometimes asked, "Aren't you disappointed, Dr. Walker, that the remedies you recommend aren't working for you?" This is a familiar question that's occasionally put to me following an illustated lecture I've just delivered on how to stop baldness and regrow hair.

To those good people who may have read what I had written and did listen to my lectures, I answer: "I do feel saddened that I didn't know of the solution to baldness at age twenty-eight when my hair problem first began to manifest itself. Just imagine how much head hair I would be displaying today at age sixty-eight if I had put my current knowledge into action during the past forty years.

"In fact," my response to the audience continues, "I have been balder, for the sparse but long grey hairs you see growing on the top of my head now are rather new. They've appeared only since my return from Germany in November 1994. It was then that I began serious research on restoring hair growth using nutritional supplementation, soybean concentrate, and a diet that encourages unwrinkled skin, firm fingernails, strong toenails, and healthy hair. Additionally, during the winter of 1995 the evidence I had accumulated overseas caused me to start utilizing the externally applied thymus gland extract and herbal solution for falling hair that I had learned about in Heidelberg, Munich, Mannheim, Darmstadt, Frankfurt, and other German cities. Oh, if only I had known forty years ago what I'm aware of today about hair loss and its regrowth."

These words which I express in replying to queries about my persistent baldness represent what I truly believe. It's obvious that most of the hair follicles on the front, top, and back of my head have died, and there is no way to restore them to life. Still, I do have new hair strands making their appearance. The individual hairs have grown over three inches long. That's because my hair follicles which were sleeping have been awakened and reactivated into growing their hairs once again. Dysfunctional dormant follicles are now stimulated into refunctioning the way nature intended them to do. I'm ever so grateful to have learned of the externally applied solution for falling hair. It's a godsend—something unexpected but particularly welcome and timely even in my advanced years!

The Externally Applied Solution for Falling Hair

In the preface, I described the cruelness of a certain barber named Antonio Sambito. Because of variations in the conditions under which adult head hair grows, flourishes, or falls out, young Thurston Clarke's clever but unfeeling school basement barber was dead wrong at that earlier time about how to stop the loss of hair and is even more incorrect today. Other than the floor, something else quite viable and practical is available to stop hair from falling further or falling at all.

There are proven methods for stopping hair loss. First and most significant is the singular method of preserving head hair with thymus gland extract derived from baby cattle. It's corrective both for men and women in their adult years. The external treatment, described in later chapters, has benefical characteristics. Regular use of the cosmetic lotion and accompanying shampoo causes particular forms of baldness to become strictly temporary and bare scalp areas do readily recover.

The same topically applied hair treatment protects the heads of cancer patients so that baldness doesn't occur from their taking necessary but cytotoxic chemotherapeutic agents. In fact, this new hair restorative was developed by German scientists at the behest of participating oncologists, gynecologists, and dermatologists administering treatment in eight German and Austrian universities. The oncological clinicians with the assistance of other researchers had been attempting to mitigate unsightly side effects that were being experienced by their cancer patients.

Today, no one need feel embarrassment or the butt of jokes as was young Thurston Clarke. There is a solution for thinning hair, falling hair, or outright baldness. Five particular items comprise the German natural hair-growing formula. They consist of a shampoo (scalp cleanser), a treatment lotion (liquid revitalizer), a hair treatment gel ("miracle grow"), a hair treatment mask (setting lotion), and the hair conditioning creme rinse. Only the first two mentioned are basic and mandatory, inasmuch as they create most of the follicular excitation.

A Natural Hair-Growing Formula

The basic hair-restoring solution is a shampoo and a lotion used in combination to stimulate the regrowth of hair strands when their hair follicles are alive. If live hair follicles are lingering inactively in the scalp or other body parts, they can give rise to new strands of hair once again. Moreover, this hair-growing solution seems to stop the white blood cells' auto-immune attack on hair follicles, which is believed by many dermatologists to be the underlying cause of an individual's hair loss.

Thymu-Skin®, the hair-growing formula, is not some magical tonic. Rather it's a stimulative natural substance possessed by every individual as a child. But it becomes much diminished or nearly lost altogether as one grows into adulthood. The natural substance is thymosin, a hormone secreted by one's thymus gland, which most people naturally have in abundance as youngsters but which is lost steadily with the advancement of age.

Combined with other herbal and nutrient ingredients, thymosin makes up much of the *Thymu-Skin®* formula that is now accessible to anyone who desires to arouse the regrowth of scalp and/or body hair. Utilizing this relatively new formulation offers anyone the ability to absorb by simple topical application an extract made from the thymus glands of calves. Simultaneous with restimulating hair growth, medical researchers postulate that it may possibly increase the number of T-lymphocytes in the bloodstream to fight off attacks by bacterial infections, toxic metals, foreign proteins, viral organisms, fungal infectors, cancer cells, and other invading pollutants attempting to break down the body's immunity. Additionally, its use may neutralize auto-immune reactions which cause components of one's body to attack another component of the body.

The newest concept in dermatology is that baldness is an autoimmune disease, one of the growing number of otherwise unrelated disorders now suspected of being caused by inflammation and destruction of tissues by the body's own antibodies—the autoantibodies. Thus, baldness has now joined other immune system dysfunctional disorders such as acquired hemolytic anemia, pernicious anemia, rheumatic fever, rheumatoid arthritis, glomerulonephritis, systemic lupus erythematosus, and several forms of thyroid dysfunction, including Hashimoto's disease. It's not known why the immune system should lose the ability to distinguish between substances that are foreign to the body and hair follicles in its own scalp. But finally we have access to a new remedy that restores recognition to attacking white blood cells so that they stop doing damage to hair follicles.

Nutrients to Stimulate Healthier Hair, Skin, and Nails

Along with health-food-store proprietors who study aspects of nutrition, physicians practicing holistic medicine are aware that deficiencies in one's diet may bring on thinning of the head hair in women (female pattern baldness) and outright baldness in men. Some nutrient manufacturers market vitamins and/or minerals formulated specifically to stimulate hair growth. Some of these formulas are available in health food stores.

The hair follicle stimulant formulas frequently contain vitamin C, the amino acid L-cysteine, and the B-complex vitamins: pare-amino benzoic acid (PABA), inositol, niacin, and biotin. All these nutrients are connected to hair growth or its coloring. For instance, the originator of orthomolecular medicine (treating illness with nutrients rather than drugs), Abram Hoffer, M.D., Ph.D., my coauthor on *Putting It All Together: The New Orthomolecular Nutrition,* reports in our book that he turned grey hair on his own chest a dark color once again by the use of niacin (vitamin B_3).[1]

In another book that we wrote together, *Smart Nutrients: A Guide to Nutrients that Can Prevent and Reverse Senility,* we say: "... one of the main functions of skin (and its outgrowths, the hair and nails), is to excrete cross-linked proteins. The body deposits in the skin [plus in the hair and nails] large molecules that cannot be excreted in the feces or in urine. Human skin grows and wears away, taking with it whatever has been deposited, in the same way that trees get rid of accumulations of minerals by shedding their leaves. . . .

"We have seen increased melanin [skin pigment] formation in patients receiving niacin—a few schizophrenics taking the vitamin noticed that their skin, especially on the flexor surfaces (under the armpit, wrist, and on an inner aspect of the elbow), turned dark brown."[2]

As with skin, the same darkening effect is exhibited with graying hair when large quantities of niacin are ingested. Over time, the hair tends to turn back to its original color. PABA has been known to reverse premature greying, too. Together, the B-vitamins, niacin, PABA, and biotin bring about a significant effect for hair rejuvenation.

Biotin is a popular nutritional for the scalp. Human bodies don't manufacture their own supply of biotin because they get enough from diets or from friendly and advantageous bacteria living in the intestines. If someone ate only egg whites or received intravenous feedings for an extended period, he or she might develop a biotin deficiency that would cause hair loss. Alopecia areata and patchy baldness do respond to the ingestion of biotin taken as a food supplement. But this B-vitamin seems to have no beneficial effect in the treatment of male pattern baldness (also known medically as *common baldness, male-pattern alopecia, androgen-dependent alopecia,* and/or *androgenetic alopecia).*

The supporters of biotin supplementation believe that it binds testosterone in the hair follicle instead of allowing this male hormone to bind with protein receptors that turn it into dihydrotestosterone (DHT). Because less DHT is availabe to "attack" the follicle, hair loss supposedly slows down or stops.

To use biotin formulas, one typically must apply biotonic conditioner once a day and pat a lotion or cream into the scalp nightly. Sometimes biotonic hair sprays for extra body in styling are recommended. Hair clinics that sell biotin treatments claim that hair stops falling after eight to ten weeks and hair growth is known to start after ten to eighteen weeks of continuous biotin therapy. The United States Food and Drug Administration (FDA) denies the effectiveness of biotin in slowing the balding process, but some users say they're happy with their results. What's needed is lots of patience and persistence when using the sprays, creams, liquids, vitamin pills and other nutritional supplements that are required as treatment.[3]

L-cysteine makes up 10 percent of the hair's protein consistency and, in laboratory experiments when taken with vitamin C, this amino acid does engender hair growth in animals being tested for certain aspects of nutrient metabolism. Whether or not they excite new hair growth, taking proteinaceous L-cysteine supplementation along with those nutrients in the vitamin B-complex plus some hair follicle stimulating minerals may be a healthy practice to pursue.

Dieting Furthers Hair Loss

The consumption of foods containing zinc is necessary to retain healthy hair. With abnormal food intake, through the use of crash dieting or from outright poverty, and drastic reduction of amounts of meat, fish, and some vegetables, zinc deficiency may set in. Then hair loss develops, and it is likely to be accompanied by diarrhea. This physical disability is followed by some psychological complications such as emotional apathy, mental confusion, and psychiatric depression. As the hair falls noticeably, abnormalities in taste and smell develop as well.

At the start of zinc deficiency, the hair becomes fine, dry, and brittle. Later it falls out in multiple strands that will be found sprinkled on the pillow. Or, it drops into the sink when washed or combed. With prolonged zinc deficiency, eczemalike scaling eruptions develop on the mouth around the lips and other mucous membranes resembling a herpes simplex viral infection. Unlike the HSV-1 infection, however, the eruptions may also occur on the arms and legs.

The treatment for zinc deficiency is simple and straightforward. Eliminate the body's starvation for minerals. Zinc supplementation has shown dramatic results in restoring the hair to its normal structure and texture; however, the best treatment is prevention by eating the foods containing elevated amounts of the mineral. Chapter Nine contains listings of foods to help maintain the proper levels of minerals required by the body.

Insufficient Biotin in the Diet

Biotin is often part of manufactured nutrient formulas touted to restore hair growth. These formulas have validity, for biotin is an essential element in fatty acid and amino acid metabolism. A diet insufficient in this vitamin may cause diffuse loss of scalp and body hair. As with zinc deficiency, lack of biotin shows an eczematoid scaling rash involving the mouth and torso. A biotin deficiency in the food supply can contribute to blurred vision, gait distrubance, muscle weakness, and tremors. Hair loss is just another manifestation of greater biotin requirements in the diet.

Unusual though it may seem, the most common reason for biotin deficiency to show up is the consumption of raw eggs, which leads to an inability of the intestine to absorb nutrients properly. The condition can also be linked to small bowel resection as occurs with surgery for inflammatory bowel disease. If nutrition is taken through a means other than the gastrointestinal tract, such as by intravenous feeding, there may be biotin deficiency. Although rare, an inherited or genetic deficiency of biotin exists.

The cure for this type of baldness or hair thinning is biotin supplementation. Biotin supplements may be acquired from almost any health food store and from many pharmacies. Better yet, eat plenty of foods containing biotin. They are listed in Chapter Nine.

Baldness from a Lack of Essential Fatty Acids

Diffuse eyebrow and scalp hair loss, and a lightening in color of the remaining hair occurs from the deficiency of essential fatty acids as part of one's daily menu. It's not uncommon to see such hair loss occur in the hospital when infants or adults remain on long-term supplemental, intravenous, or tube-administered feedings. This type of therapeutic nutrition may result in an absence of certain fatty acids from the parenteral fluid. It's an error that lies squarely on the shoulders of a careless hospital dietitian. Added to one's loss of hair from insufficient intake of essential fatty acids may be dry, scaling eruptions of the skin folds that resembles eczema—the same as in zinc and/or biotin deficiencies.

Here, too, the treatment is easy to apply by restoring linoleic acid in the form of flax seeds and safflower oil (which is 65 percent linoleic acid) to the food supply. New hair growth and healing of the skin lesions follows treatment, often as quickly as a few weeks.

Iron Deficiency Causes Hair Loss

For women with thinning hair or outright alopecia, iron deficiency, even in the absence of anemia, could be responsible for their condition. The well-known iron-deficiency anemia is one of the more common causes of diffuse hair loss for older women. Consequently, hair mineral analysis and iron blood levels should be tested in all women with nonscarring hair loss.

Hair regrowth can occur rapidly when nutritional supplements containing iron are utilized on a daily basis. The ingrowth of new hair usually begins three to six months after the program of supplementation commences.

Weight Reduction Diets May Cause Hair Loss

Someone who engages in overly enthusiastic dieting for purposes of achieving a serious weight reduction is liable to experience hair loss as well. Falling hair shows itself about three months after strict dieting to decrease the total body weight by 15 to 20 percent. Bariatricians who treat obese people look for that type of hair loss and are known to have their patients taper off in their dieting when it happens.

Blood loss, including the voluntary donation of blood to the Red Cross or at a local hospital, may also contribute to falling hair. In that case, ridding the body of iron from the bloodstream may be the culprit for causing hair to fall.

In both food deprivation and blood loss, the attendant hair loss is likely to be a consequence of the reduction of proteins necessary for hair to grow. For most people who resume proper nutritional intake, however, the hair growth will restore itself in three to twelve months following that person's termination of the initial acute assault on his or her body.[4]

American men spend more than $1.2 billion per year on hair-loss treatments.[5] Until now, following my abandoning the wearing of hair pieces thirty years ago, I've not been one of them. Quite simply, I had accepted my baldness as nonreversible. It's well known that most hair growing remedies are ineffective and do not work. But my opinion was totally changed as a result of those observations I made in Germany during the autumn of 1994. Results for hair follicle stimulation were excellent then, and they're even better today. I am using the remedies recommended here and so does Jules, the youngest of my three sons to whom I've dedicated this book. By acting on what you'll learn in the following chapters, my prediction is that you'll count yourself fortunate in having acquired *Bald No More: How to Stop Baldness and Regrow Hair.*

CHAPTER ONE

Psychological Aspects of Losing Your Hair

Baldness can present a serious social embarrassment to a man and, more especially to a woman. It inevitably adds years to the individual's general physical appearance. In today's fashion-conscious society, many people choose to hide their baldness by taking one, two, or more of the following actions: wearing a hairpiece, taking nutritional supplements and herbal remedies, performing scalp massage, undergoing hair replacement surgeries, accepting hair weaves, rubbing in colored potions smelling of tar, sitting under buzzing metal contraptions to stimulate hair follicles with electricity, and trying other methods to make head hair return or to preserve what is left.

I was one of those people who, having begun balding noticeably at age twenty-eight, started looking around for some means of holding onto my remaining dark brown, thick and curly locks.

From eight years old onward, I used a steel-toothed animal comb for flattening my mop of abundantly knotted hair. I remember, I often looked at myself in the mirror and wished for those thickly packed curls to disappear. I wanted them to become thin and straight hair strands, looking like everyone else's. Or, I thought, at least there could be fewer of those overabundant ringlets. Well, I rapidly had my wish fulfilled. Today at sixty-eight, I am quite bald!

I came to accept the wearing of a toupee (hairpiece) daily for two years starting in 1967 to cover a condition of male pattern baldness advancing steadily across my pate. In those days I practiced in Stamford, Connecticut as a licensed foot specialist (Doctor of Podiatric Medicine) who sat at people's feet performing procedures to provide my patients with foot comfort.

The early March day that I first walked out of the hairpiece shop in New York City wearing that dark, silky, and skull-cap-like toupee was devastating for me. That's because to attach the piece firmly onto my scalp, any remaining hair strands growing in patches atop my head needed to be removed. The wig shop's barber had run his electric razor around the top of my noggin as if it was a lawn needing mowing. When he was done, the shop's mirror seemed to reflect a Byzantine monk with a circle of bareness exposing a very white scalp! When previously it had been usual for me to delude myself with the sparse but observable hairs growing on top, now I truly was committed to covering my baldness with the newly acquired wig.

Faithfully each morning, I pasted that hairpiece to my scalp using double-backed adhesive tape. Each night before slipping beneath the covers, I was equally dutiful about dissolving off the residue of sticky adhesive with benzene. My wife objected at first to the benzene odor in bed, but it was one of the requirements Joan faced in order to stay happily married to me.

Those returning foot care patients who hadn't visited my office for a long time would ask, "Dr. Walker, have you lost weight? There's something different about you!" Often I agreed to the weight loss theory. Foot sufferers who consulted me monthly never mentioned the obvious change in my appearance, except they always seemed to be looking at the top of my head. Sometimes I'd overhear whispered discussions among the patients and my podiatric assistants: "Don't say anything!" was the employees' official advice.

Lots of funny stories (embarrassing at the time) might be told about my experiences with the toupee. One of those hair-raising tales involved the time I had been participating in a judo contest during May of 1967. I should mention that the manner in which I showed my head to viewers was a perpetual source of stress to me and always required some advance planning.

With this particular judo match, my pride (or vanity, if you prefer) didn't allow me to appear in public wearing my white quilted judo gee with my green belt, and showing my totally bald head. I had an image to uphold among friends, neighbors, and patients of mine who were members of the audience. Remember that my head under the hairpiece was shaved cleanly around the forehead, crown, and rear so that the double-back adhesive tape would have scalp on which to stick and not slide on loose hairs. I wore my hairpiece as an integral part of the image I presented to the public.

From one corner of the mat, my opponent (an expert Japanese brown belt judo player who was surely going to beat me) approached and made stabbing motions at my gee collar with his clawed fingers. Either of us would take hold of any part of the opponent's anatomy that became exposed— arms, legs, etc. He struck first and grabbed for my head to cup it between both his hands and pull me down into a headlock. Consequently, "the tranch" (my young sons compared the fake hair's furry look and feel to that of a tarantula) came off in my opponent's hands. This brown belt player became so confused by my sliding out from under his grasp while he still held onto a piece of my head that the puzzled fellow was easily thrown to the mat. Almost under false pretenses, I won the judo match. My sensei (judo teacher) and the audience laughed and laughed.

Then there's the time I was swimming laps on a hot August day in 1968. It was at our suburban area's community swimming pool. Upon turning to repeat my swim strokes down the long lap line, I bumped into my tranch floating on top of the water. After that, I was the only man in Stamford, Connecticut who swam wearing a woman's bathing cap.

For the previous nine years I had strictly driven sporty convertibles, which caused my fellow foot health professionals to name me "Mort the Sport." It was my joy to roll along on a warm spring day with the car top down and the wind whistling past my ears. Upon the advent of my hairpiece, driving with the top up, no matter how sunny and hot the weather, became an absolute rigid rule for me. Eventually I sold those sporty convertibles and bought a sedan with airconditioning.

All such circumstances involving the toupee ended when during a routine physical examination my longstanding friend and personal physician, Ezra Epstein, M.D., discovered me wearing the beanie-like item made from another person's dark brown hair. He grabbed the toupee off my head and asked, "What's this, a rug? Why don't you get rid of the thing and just grow old gracefully?" Several months later, I took Dr. Epstein's advice. Being totally uneducated about hair growth and its loss, I didn't know what else to do except accept my fate as an old baldy.

Dr. Aldhizer Experiences Depression from His Baldness

My experience with baldness and attempts at its repair, of course, are not uncommon. Fifty-four-year-old T. Gerard Aldhizer, M.D., a graduate of the Medical College of Virginia, who practices family medicine in Richmond, Virginia, tells the story of emotional involvement with his own baldness. From age thirty, Dr. Aldhizer had been bald, and he was very unhappy with his condition. He was so emotionally depressed by baldness that he tried all types of techniques to make head hair grow or give the appearance that it was on top when there really wasn't anything much there at all.

Dr. Aldhizer confesses in *The Doctor's Book on Hair Loss,* that he doesn't like "Bald." Bald was the enemy he and I have battled, tried to deceive, and continued to wage war on since the fateful day, when at thirty, his father welcomed him to The Club. His hair loss started in the front, meaning the whole front: the left side, the right side, and the middle. Just discharged from U.S. Navy medical service, Dr. Aldhizer was practicing medicine in Richmond, Virginia and trying to rebuild a social life that had been bombed by the military service.

When the doctor first noticed his hairline was receding, he took the situation calmly. "It's bound to be a slow process. Probably won't change my appearance for years and years," Dr. Aldhizer said to himself. But his mirror told him otherwise. He was beginning to lose hair at an alarming rate. It was leaving fast enough to require some action.

Having always parted his hair on the right, his first tactic was to let that side grow longer and comb those long hairs across the bald spot. He used a squirt or two of hair spray to hold the hairs in place. Each shot of spray became instant self-confidence. He could still walk up to a mirror and see an attractive person. "There was still a bounce in my walk," he said. "Then Bald really mobilized. Soon I wasn't just bare along the front; I was bare on the top."

Dr. Aldhizer geared up—the part became lower and the hair grew longer. Much longer. He loaded his arsenal with cans of hair spray and advanced from a couple of squirts per grooming to a quarter of a can or more. The amount depended on the activity planned. A quarter of a can was fine for the office and patients. Anything else and the stock in Clairol [a hair-preparation company] shot through the roof. For example, if he planned to be outside and a wind was blowing, it was half a can. For a date that included dancing, half a can at intervals. The amount of spray used became directly proportionate to the amount of activity anticipated. It was not a formula he had learned in medical school, but it was a formula that kept him active. Dr. Aldhizer was still able to face himself in the mirror—but there wasn't a lot of bounce in his walk.

At the time he didn't realize he had entered the first serious phase of warfare against Bald—The Big Wrap-Over (The Big Wrap, for short). His part was only a few centimeters above his right ear and his hair on the right side was as long as it would grow. He had switched from mild hair sprays to canned concrete—the heaviest and the thickest stuff on the market. He wasn't bouncing now, and started seeing a hairstylist.

Dr. Aldhizer points out that there were three enemies of his Big Wrap: wind, water, and women. Wind made the hair that he combed sideways across his head blow out from the side like a flapping flag. He avoided wind at all costs or wore a hat even on the hottest days. Water had his Big Wrap hair floating to the surface like so many snakes; subsequently, he gave up swimming which he loved. And the single women he dated became most dangerous when they persisted in running their fingers through the Big Wrap. Many a relationship was ruined when a woman slid her hand under the long combed and sprayed hairs he had so carefully pasted down so that his bare scalp became revealed. Then he knew that she knew with certainty about his baldness and he felt compelled to sever the relationship. The knowledge that a woman knew, caused Dr. Aldhizer to feel self-conscious, sense his inadequateness, and fall even deeper into depression.

"I had used the Big Wrap and untold cans of hair spray. I tried sutures and a hairpiece. I let my head be bombarded with synthetic fibers. The membership card (in the baldness club) seemed indestructible. Getting out of The Club was tougher than getting out of the military," he confessed.

To leave the baldness club and fool himself with the delusion of joining the ranks of men having full heads of hair, Dr. Aldhizer started wearing a hairpiece in 1983. In reality, however, he remained bald and possibly continues to be emotionally involved with his hair loss even today. His book, published in 1983, needs a sequel to tell the rest of this sad but true bald-headed tale.[1]

The doctor's story about his baldness is available to the public. It's a tale with which all of us old baldies—especially single males who are dating and seeking a mate—may identify. Dr. Aldhizer's description is amusing but it's rife with emotionalism as well.

Balding Women Become Even More Emotional

Hair loss can be particularly traumatic when it affects women, even though it is a relatively common condition. As I previously discussed, thinning hair or outright baldness can be triggered by particular factors in one's metabolism such as crash diets, medications, stress, childbirth, or nutritional deficiencies. But often it seems to happen for no apparent reason at all.[2]

About two out of three women residing in Western industrialized countries suffer temporary or permanent hair loss at some time in life.[3] And over 60 percent of all women worldwide begin to experience some hair loss by the time they reach menopause.[4]

Every day is a bad hair day for those 21 million American women who suffer from degrees of baldness. Endlessly fussing with wigs, hair additions, and hats, with little satisfaction, many have said they feel like less of a woman, often choose jobs that keep them out of the public eye. Sometimes women suffering from hair loss come down with psychosomatic illnesses. All levels of society recognizes that hair is a clear sign of female sexuality, and it's unquestioned that women who lose their hair tend to believe that they are devalued in some way. They can feel pain and despair, and some even become suicidal, as was the experience for Karen Renken who, as Dr. Aldhizer had done, put her baldness story into print.

A Sad Hair Story

Hair loss is a nightmare for anyone, but for Karen Renken it was unspeakably horrid. She told her story in *Cosmopolitan* magazine. Karen, who exemplifies a type of woman affected by the tendency to hair loss, first noticed herself balding when she was only seventeen. Her hair's thinness followed a haircut given by her girlfriend who was not a hairdresser. Her friend botched the job, and to fix it Karen visited the local hair salon, where she to received another, even shorter, haircut.

Karen wrote that it seemed to take forever to grow back, and because it was in short layers. She noticed her scalp was showing through in certain areas. Her part was widening, and strands of hair fell out whenever she combed it.''

A dermatologist Karen consulted advised that her thinning hair came from the often hereditary condition, androgenetic alopecia, (the commonly known male/female pattern baldness). The dermatologist administered chemicals and ultraviolet light to her head for a few minutes. The teenager also received prescriptions for a special shampoo, cortisone medicinal scalp cream to apply nightly, and a supply of B-complex vitamins such as biotin and niacin to be swallowed each day in hopes of growing hair.

Anxious to see results, Karen rushed to the mirror every morning, searching for improvement, but was disappointed every day. After several months, she stopped the treatments and decided to try a perm. At first it worked well, but eventually it only made her condition worse.

Another dermatologist she consulted was convinced hormone imbalance was the culprit responsible for Karen's hair loss. He sent her for laboratory tests and declared that if the hair follicles weren't dead, medication would correct the problem. The prescriptions did not work, and she progressed further into baldness.

At the age of eighteen, the unfortunate woman contemplated suicide over her ordeal. She was still trying to cover up the hair loss by constantly combing my hair over the thin areas.'' One night, Karen's new boyfriend Jimmy said jokingly, 'if you don't stop combing your hair, it will fall out altogether.' She started crying and explained the situation to him. He was very sweet and understanding—but she lost him.

As her hair loss got progressively worse, she dreaded going to the beauty parlor. The walk from the shampoo sink to the haircutter's chair seemed to take an eternity for her. There was no way she could cover up the baldness when her hair was wet. (She had ceased going swimming with her friends for the same reason.) As Karen became more self-conscious, she spent a fortune on hair products such as thickeners, sprays, special shampoos and anything else she thought would help. Whenever she saw a woman (or man) with beautiful hair, Karen felt pangs of envy.

Hair-loss woes contributed to her gaining weight. As she became despondent over her appearance, she turned to eating for solace. It became a vicious cycle: getting depressed, binging, then getting more depressed. In her mid-twenties, one hundred pounds overweight, with hair so thin that everyone stared, Karen Renken's self-esteem could not have gone any lower.

While this woman did manage to deal with her weight-gain problem effectively by using a stringent diet and fitness training to drop the hundred pounds over a year's time, she couldn't find any permanent hair-growing solution. Instead, Karen resorted to hair weaving as the masking method for covering up her baldness. Hair weaving is a technique of braiding one's remaining real hair and then sewing, taping or snapping into it a wig comprised of somebody else's extra hair or synthetic fibers (see Chapter Ten). This attached wig is the equivalent of a man's hairpiece only the hair weave gets blended into the more abundant remaining growth that a woman might have left to her.[5]

Psychological Consequences of Baldness

For a manly man, there probably was a time when he was most proud of his hair—maybe as a twenty-eight-year-old, which had been my own situation. During an earlier time his hair might have been mousseable, featherable, fluffable, gelable, spikeable—a real sprouting bush atop his head. This hair had attitude. It said to the world "I am handsome, youthful, potent, physical, and full of vitally. Most of all, I am not bald!"

It was a statement a man was proud to make—until lately, for disaster has struck. Those twin horseshoes of new forehead above the temples have made themselves apparent, along with that gravity-prone flatness at the crown, known to dermatologists as "the vertex balding pattern." Finally there shows a burgeoning Friar Tuck white space around the back of the head which declares to everyone making eye contact that a man is undergoing the acknowledged tragedy of male-pattern baldness (MPB).[6]

For men with the vertex balding pattern, the psychological consequences of baldness have yet to be uncovered. It may be the reason that Trappist monasteries have become so popular as refuges of meditation, prayer, and retreat.

As reported by *America On-Line:* it's been established that 25 percent of bald men would trade five years of life for a full head of hair. The alopecia has them psychologically debilitated. A full, thick head of hair is such a powerful symbol of youth and attractiveness that its absence is absolutely devastating.[7]

The American Hair Loss Council (AHLC) in Schaumburg, Illinois advises that hair loss has varying negative effects on one's self-consciousness and self-esteem, depending upon an individual's personality, sex, age, and marital status. Those who suffer from the condition typically feel anxious and embarrassed about their hair loss because they are so obviously impacted physically, yet feel helpless to prevent it.

"The psychological implications are obvious when you see how sensitive male and female patients can be about their hair loss," says Maureen McKeown, a hair restoration medical assistant. "The loss of control is often more than they can take, to the point of paranoia about anyone touching the hair that remains or suicidal tendencies because they feel they simply don't look 'normal' anymore."

The problem hits men particularly hard as it strikes at the age most are trying to advance in their careers and social lives, and because their alternatives for camouflaging hair loss are limited.

Still, loss of hair is even more demolishing to women's psyches, because so many believe they are freakish. They look at their bald heads in mirrors and see anomalies that keep them feeling uncomfortable with themselves throughout each day. In addition, female pattern baldness (FPB) had been more difficult to treat because it shows up as a diffuse thinning of hair across the scalp. This is in contrast to identifiable areas of baldness observable in men. (See Chapter Two.)

"Patients that enter our hair restoration office often are visibly bothered by their appearance and obviously are in psychological pain," says Ms. McKeown. "Many times they have suffered teasing by others, but are still hardest on themselves."

"The failure and/or limitations of temporary topical products like minoxidil (Rogaine®), coupled with the already low self-esteem associated with hair loss, only compounds the impact of balding on all aspects of the lives of the many sufferers—especially with regard to patients' psychological, social, and emotional well-being," adds Robert Leonard, immediate past president of the International Society of Hair Restoration Surgery (ISHRS), also located in Schaumburg, Illinois.

As part of its public information program, the AHLC tells us that people between the ages of eighteen and twenty-nine are the most motivated to seek treatment for hair loss. Of the 65 million American men and women affected by baldness, 17.5 percent seek help of some kind either by health professional care, barbershop and/or beauty salon advice, or from use of over-the-counter remedies to achieve hair follicle stimulation for the establishment of hair strand regrowth. The American Hair Loss Council reiterates that key factors leading sufferers to seek treatment include feeling a loss of control over aging and mortality, a decline in self-confidence, and a desire to feel better equipped professionally and socially.

MPB Adversely Affects the Psychology of Some Men

From the Department of Psychology at Old Dominion University in Norfolk, Virginia, Thomas F. Cash, Ph.D., reports on possible psychological effects created in men by the appearance of baldness. From his published clinical journal article, **Table 1-1**, divided into "low-hair-loss," and "high-hair-loss," lists what Dr. Cash found as some of the most salient effects of hair loss reported by balding men. Male pattern baldness has an adverse, stressful impact on most men but does not alter the personality functioning of the majority of them. High-hair-loss men had greater overall body image dissatisfaction than nonbalding control subjects. Those balding men younger than age twenty-six reported the most intense preoccupation and coping efforts in response to their hair loss.[8]

TABLE 1–1

Percentage of Men Attributing Specific Psychological Effects to the Occurrence of Male Pattern Baldness (MPB)

Reported Experience	Extent of Hair Loss	
	Low Loss	High Loss
Wish for more hair	52	84
Notice other bald/balding men	54	82
Spend much time viewing own head in mirrors	54	69
Wonder what others think about baldness	47	67
Receive excessive teasing from peers	45	79

Feel self-conscious about hair's appearance	42	78
Look older than actual age	40	55
Worry that others will notice the baldness	39	56
Feel helpless about the presence of MPB	37	56
Feel anxiety about aging prematurely	37	46
Feel less attractive because of MPB	31	51
Envy good-looking, bushy-haired men	33	34
Trying to improve hairstyle to hide baldness	63	66
Trying to improve physique to offset baldness	41	36
Dresses with more attention to clothes because of MPB	26	45
Wears hats or caps more often as part of ensemble	23	41
Seeks reassurance from friends about looks	23	39
Grew a beard or mustache to offset baldness	18	36

Our culture places a premium on physical appearance, and conditions like male pattern baldness can have an adverse effect on the psyche. Contrary to prevalent assumptions that only women have body-image problems, Dr. Cash's findings implicate MPB as contributing to men's body-image concerns. Still, the psychological effects of female pattern baldness or other forms of alopecia on women are likely to be even more deleterious than those observed among men, a second hypothesis Dr. Thomas Cash investigated in August 1991.[9]

The Shame and Grief of Baldness

Unreported in the psychological or dermatological literature is that many men and women who are just beginning
to experience hair loss go into a state of denial. Then, when
complete baldness overcomes them, they look into the mirror
and say, "that's not me," knowing full well that "bad hair
days" or rather "no hair days" are their destiny. That isn't
the situation for Martha Chiarapa anymore, who revealed
her alopecia areata in a personal narrative told in the June
1996 issue of the *Ladies Home Journal*.

During late spring 1981, her husband, Richard Chiarapa,
noticed a tiny bare spot on the top of his wife's head, and
both of them laughed at his remark when he joked, "I always
thought I'd be the one to go bald." The mother of two
daughters aged four and six, Martha Chiarapa at thirty-three,
possessed thick, reddish brown hair and pursued her full-
time occupation as a homemaker in suburban Hartford, Connecticut.

When in mid-September the little bald spot had grown to
the size of a quarter, Mrs. Chiarapa consulted a dermatologist
who immediately diagnosed her hair problem as a form of
alopecia areata that not only causes loss of hair on the scalp
but also over the balance of the body. Specifically, she was
the victim of *alopecia universalis et totalis* (see Chapter
Two.) "You could lose the whole crown," the doctor told
her matter-of-factly. "Just put a wig on your head and a
smile on your face."

Within weeks the woman permanently lost huge tufts out
of her scalp, and reddish brown hair fell onto her shoulders
like dead needles from a diseased pine tree. Her eyelashes
fell off and her eyebrows came out. The dermatologist treated
Mrs. Chiarapa with a variety of drugs, including cortisone
(steroid) creams, cortisone injections, oral Prednisone®
(another steroid), and numbers of different additional prescriptions. For her, a main adverse side effect of the Predni-
sone® was mental and emotional depression. None of the
prescriptions worked, and the only way Martha Chiarapa

could "self-treat" her disability was to cover it with a bandanna at first and then later a wig.

She still wears wigs, but now they're more expensive ones ranging in cost from $1,600 to $3,000, which Mrs. Chiarapa gets from an Australian company. The wig is attached to a custom-fit fiber-glass cap that suctions firmly onto the head. She's become one of the company's more successful wig distributors in the U.S.A.[10]

Mrs. Martha Chiarapa, Ms. Karen Renken, and Dr. T. Gerald Aldhizer have all resorted to using wigs as a means of covering their baldness. Unfortunately for them, sufficient scientific information had failed to traverse the Atlantic Ocean into the United States from Germany advising that a new, naturally-occurring, hair-growing preparation processed from calf thymus and combined with various herbal, nutritional, and pharmaceutical ingredients is available. This advanced product under the carefully selected brand name *Thymu-Skin*® works effectively for several specific types of hair loss, though not for all types.

One wonders if Mrs. Chiarapa or Ms. Renken or Dr. Aldhizer's balding problem would respond to topical applications of the new remedy. The only way to answer such a question for them or somebody else is by a product trial. Alternatively, knowing in advance what is the source of one's hair loss and why it has developed could possibly preclude any unrewarding investment of time, money, and anticipation. The next chapter will discuss various kinds of baldness and propose known reasons for their manifestations.

CHAPTER TWO

What Baldness Is and Why It Develops

At age twenty-six, Phillip Morlock of Toronto, a printer's apprentice, went through his personal period of emotional devastation when Sarah Valentine, the girl whom he was proposing to marry, broke off their relationship. The tragedy happened simply because it appeared that Phillip was going to look like his very bald father. In contrast, this ex-girlfriend's own dad possessed hair as thick and tight as a Berber rug, and she admired her father.

Because their meetings had been mostly at night in parked cars, darkened taverns, poorly lit social gatherings or in dim restaurants, Sarah had not noticed that the top of Phillip's scalp held a small pancake-size patch of bareness. One evening, before he took the opportunity to propose marriage, Sarah ran her fingers through Phil's hair and stopped in midstroke. She had found the bald spot. Directly after that, she dropped him, and, unfortunately, was honest enough to tell the heartbroken fellow why. Looking to the future, Sarah had said, "I just can't see myself with a bald boyfriend." Little did she know that it had been his intention to make himself her bald husband.

The Long and Short of Hair Growth

In the fairy tale, when Rapunzel let down her hair from the tower in which she was imprisoned for the prince to climb up, she had no clue that a genetic defect probably lay at the root of her golden locks. But a 1994 experiment in developmental biology conducted at the University of California, San Francisco, revealed that the presence of a growth factor—contrary to its name—limits the length that hair will grow. "When the factor is missing, hair grows very, very long," reported Gail L. Martin, Ph.D., a biologist working in laboratories at that west coast university.

Along with other researchers, Dr. Martin was studying a chemical messenger called *fibroblast growth factor 5* in mice that lacked the gene for this particular messenger. The scientists were observing how its loss would affect embryonic development. To their surprise, the newborn mice looked and acted normal—at least at first. But a few weeks after their birth Dr. Martin and her colleagues noticed that the young mice with missing growth factor looked a bit shaggy. Their hair grew longer than what was usual for baby mice.

Normally, hair grows in cycles. First, a hair follicle develops. Deep inside it lies a bud of mesodermal tissue which causes the bud to divide and sprout as a hair. Eventually, it stops growing. The follicle becomes quiescent, and the hair falls out so that the cycle can begin again.

Dr. Martin's research group's genetic analyses indicate that a known abnormal factor called *the angora gene* is actually a variant of the gene for this growth factor. She says that people, too, may have the angora variant. According to her concept, fibroblast growth factor 5 is the first, but probably not the only, chemical signal discovered for the hair cycle. "There's obviously a backup signal, because the hair doesn't grow forever," she noted during her presentation to the annual meeting of the Society for Cell Biology, that was held in San Francisco.[1]

There is no greater right-between-the-eyes reminder that youth is checking out—leaving no forwarding address—

than the first time you see a drain clogged with your own hair. There are many different forms of baldness which could require defensive actions.

The Numerous Forms of Baldness

Baldness, referred to by the medical profession as *alopecia,* is the partial or complete loss of hair from the head or the body or both. It may result from a genetic trait, systemic disease, hormonal defect, drug side effect, aging, anticancer treatment, skin disorder, another systemic source, or from some local cause. Numerous forms of this condition exist, and in this chapter various medical definitions are offered, and these same descriptive terms will be referred to in later chapters. Here are examples of the more common baldness conditions:

In *alopecia areata,* there are well-defined bald patches, often round or oval in shape. They present themselves on the head, beard, and other hairy parts of the body. Even if the condition clears up within a year without treatment, it's common for the suddenly visible alopecia areata to recur somewhat later. A few other less common names are used to identify this problem too. It's variably called *alopecia celsi, alopecia circumscripta,* and *Jonston's alopecia.*

Quite often the *alopecia areata* condition responds well to the hair revitalizing ingredient in *Thymu-Skin®,* which reactivates dormant hair follicles in men and women, revitalizes normal hair cells for fuller, thicker, healthier hair, and is applicable with positive results in almost all cases of thinning hair for both genders. If a full program of *Thymu-Skin®* is applied, the *alopecia areata* does not return.

Alopecia universalis is a complete loss of hair from all parts of the body. It sometimes occurs as an extension of generalized alopecia areata, and *Thymu-Skin®* frequently *does* work well to correct this condition.

In *patchy alopecia* ("patchy" is only a descriptive term), areas develop on the parietal (front) and occipital (back) regions of the scalp that look moth-eaten. The condition is suspected of being connected with the invasion of some microorganism inasmuch as such hair loss has occasionally been a secondary characteristic of various infections. Dr. Klio Moessler, one of the main dermatologists at the Dermatological Department of the Municipal Clinics of Darmstadt in Germany, who participated in research on diseases producing baldness and new potential hair-growing products, points out, "Patchy alopecia may come from a fungal or bacterial infection or from genetic defects involving the hair. It occurs in cicatricial (scar-forming) alopecia, alopecia areata, and some skin diseases." *Thymu-Skin®* may not be effective in treating some of the more complicated causes of patchy alopecia.

For *alopecia totalis* (complete baldness), all the hair on the scalp is lost. This is an uncommon head hair defect with no known cause, but it does respond to the calf thymus preparation described in this book.

With the three types of *alopecia areatas (patchy, universalis, and totalis)* evidence is mounting that an immunological signal is involved. (See Chapter Five.) In the double condition diagnosed as *alopecia areata totalis et universalis,* the entire head and body of an individual becomes bald. Hair disappears from the pubic region, armpits, eyelashes, eyebrows, chest, legs, beard, and other areas. It has been proven in clinical studies that *Thymu-Skin®* is useful in reversing the effects of the combination condition of *alopecia areata totalis et universalis* as well.

Baldness has traditionally been considered to be irreversible, without any corrective treatment—before today. Immunological aspects of alopecia will be discussed at length in Chapters Eleven and Twelve.

In *alopecia disseminata,* also referred to as *alopecia diffusa,* there is hair loss around the whole scalp or even from all other parts of the body. The cause may be a nutritional deficiency (especially lack of zinc or iron), a dysfunction of the thyroid gland, a polluting intoxicant, or some chronic and generalized illness. *Alopecia diffusa* can't be corrected with *Thymu-Skin®* unless the underlying difficulty is found and eliminated.

As regarding *alopecia androgenetica* (also known in dermatology as *alopecia hereditaria)*, approximately half of the adult males residing in the United States and other Western industrialized countries exhibit this condition. Dr. Moessler told me that at least 65 percent of all German men suffer from the problem. In men, some of the other names for the condition of alopecia androgenetica are *male pattern baldness, androgenetic alopecia, premature baldness, seborrheic alopecia, common baldness, hereditary baldness.* In women, *alopecia androgenetica* is referred to as *female pattern baldness* or *diffuse alopecia.* (See the accompanying patterns of androgenetic alopecia in **Drawing 5-1** and **Drawing 5-2** for men and women in Chapter 5.)

Rodney Dawber, M.A., M.B., Ch.B., who is consulting dermatologist at the Churchill Hospital in Oxford and clinical senior lecturer in dermatology at Oxford University, both in the United Kingdom, and Dominique Van Neste, M.D., Ph.D., Director of the Skin Study Center in Tournai, Belgium, have joined together to declare: ''Androgenetic alopecia probably occurs to a degree in all adults some time after puberty—only being obvious in some women in old age.''[2]

Dermatologists, both in the United States and in Europe, strongly suspect the loss of hair arises from a baldness gene which men and/or women with *androgenetic alopecia* inherit from their fathers and occasionally from their mothers.

The Conjectured Reason for Androgenetic Alopecia

But with all the conjecture among hair specialists, the true reason for *alopecia androgenetica* to occur is not entirely known. Dermatologists do recognize that it is the most common form of baldness showing up in males and females. Its onset happens at puberty in genetically predisposed individuals, and the condition is an autosomal dominant disorder.[3] Autosomal dominant refers to a pattern of inheritance in which a dominant gene on a nonsex determining chromosome (the autosome) makes a certain characteristic of a disorder. Individuals affected with *alopecia androgenetica* usually have a bald parent. However, normal children of the affected parent do not carry the baldness trait. Thus, among two male siblings having a bald father, one son may be bald and the other not. The nonbald brother will not pass on the autosome for baldness to his sons or daughters, but the bald brother may do so.

Idiopathic male/female pattern baldness is a separate condition, too. The term, *idiopathic,* means that the medical profession acknowledges that it has not yet determined the cause of this form of baldness.

To clarify what's been stated about hereditary baldness, in *alopecia androgenetica* or *alopecia hereditaria,* the male pattern baldness and female pattern forms result from sex-influenced dominant inheritance. Androgen (meaning *hormonal* stimulation is required to produce hair loss in heterozygous individuals (in which there are two different genes situated at the same place on matched chromosomes). For example, the individual with male pattern baldness could have inherited the bald-headed gene from one parent (mother or father) and the alternative gene from the other parent. The offspring (boy or girl) of a heterozygous carrier of the bald-headed gene has a 50 percent chance of inheriting this hair-loss gene from his or her parent. There is a relationship of androgenetic alopecia and increased circulating androgens, at puberty, which probably represents one of the precipitating events in such a heterogeneous hair disorder.[4]

Furthermore, the cause of androgenetic alopecia appears to be related mostly to androgen metabolism in the skin, the hair follicle, and the sebaceous gland lobule. Hair scientists have found hormonal abnormalities of cytosol and nuclear cell receptors and cytoplasmic-carrying proteins and minerals, especially within the body's metabolism of calcium and iron.[5]

Underlying Sources of Baldness

Biology and body chemistry gone awry together and simultaneously are the usual causes of baldness, particularly in men but also in those women who may possess too much testosterone—the male hormone. In that case, a woman could be exhibiting female pattern baldness (FPB) by her hair's obvious thinning as a result of chronic loss caused by an excess of male hormone being generated by her endocrine system.

Male pattern baldness most likely starts with testosterone, the hormone produced in the testes that helps make a man a man. Testosterone is a naturally occurring hormone that stimulates the growth of male (androgen) characteristics. As testosterone throbs through the body, it interacts with an enzyme called 5-alpha reductase, which is concentrated in a man's genitals and skin. The enzyme converts testosterone into a more potent hormone called dihydrotestosterone (DHT), which some urologists have referred to as "testosterone times ten." It is formed directly from testosterone in tissue, particularly in the secondary sex organs and is highly biologically active (except in muscle and bone). DHT is necessary for male external genital development, such as the formation of the penis, scrotum, and prostate.

In the scalp, each hair follicle is genetically programmed to react differently to DHT. Men with MPB have DHT-sensitive follicles at the front or top of their heads, which wither and die from extended exposure to the hormone. It stands to reason that the onset of balding might be prevented biologically by one of several strategies:

A. By stopping the body's production of testosterone.
B. By stopping the testosterone from becoming DHT.
C. By blocking DHT before it gets to follicles.
D. By making follicles less sensitive to DHT.

A man interested in curing his baldness would probably skip strategy A, because it involves castration at an early age. Eunuchs never go bald. Although the German scientists who have perfected the hair-growing qualities of the calf-derived product, *Thymu-Skin®*, don't exactly know how it works, they believe it does accomplish at least one of the remaining B, C, or D strategies, or all three, or just two of the three. Perhaps strategy D is the most logical explanation of the product's action: making follicles less vulnerable to hormonal ravages.

In Chapter Eleven, I'll be presenting a fifth highly significant strategy showing that *Thymu-Skin®* modifies one's overactive immune system function. Manfred Hagedorn, M.D., chief of Dermatology at the Municipal Clinics of Darmstadt, points out that baldness has been shown under the microscope to be an auto-immune disease wherein one's leucocytes consisting of lymphocytes and macrophages actually attack hair follicles and cause them to go into dormancy.

In *alopecia androgenica,* another separate disease, a male-type baldness associated with excessive endocrine gland (androgenic) activity prevails in women as well. This specifically female condition, labelled above as FPB, is similar to *alopecia androgenetica.* It has a *genetic* background coming under the influence of androgen hormones in which the woman possesses more testosterone than she needs.

Chapter Thirteen includes the first clinical study conducted by Prof. Dr. Hagedorn and Dr. Moessler who utilized the new German hair-growing product and produced a reversal of *alopecia androgenetica* in 67 percent of men and 100 percent of women participating in their investigation. Also the two dermatologists carried out a second clinical study that demonstrated the regrowth of hair from the application of *Thymu-Skin®* for 43 percent of participating bald men and 94 percent of bald women.

It's Usual to Be Confused by Baldness Terminology

The lines of differentiation in internal medicine, plastic surgery, and dermatology regarding differences in these various baldness conditions are not clearcut. Many physicians have their own problems with diagnosing the reason for scalp disorders. As an example of the massive confusion in the subject, one notes that the medical textbook, *Disorders of Hair Growth: Diagnosis and Treatment,* distinguishes among several hundred types of individual hair losses occurring from diseases, disorders, or deficiencies.[6] Here is a list of just a few of them taken from another dermatology textbook:[7]

Lupus erythematosus	Childbirth, postpartum period
Lichen planus pilaris	Episodes of fever
Planopilaris	Surgery
Pseudopelade	Drugs
Scleroderma	Endocrinopathies e.g. excess androgen
Bullous pemphigoid	Nutritional metabolic disorders
Epidermolysis bullosa acquista	Autoimmune diseases
Folliculitis secondary to infection	Chemical and physical damage
Granulomatous inflammation	Nonscarring pseudopelade
Benign neoplasms	Malignant tumors
Ichthyosis congenita	Hair traction from styling
Seborrheic dermatitis	Follicular mucinosis

During my recent appearance as the guest expert on a radio talk show in Vancouver, British Columbia, Canada I was discussing hair loss. A program caller quizzed me and then stated, ''I know why men go bald. They wear hats that cut off their blood circulation and prevent the scalp from 'breathing.' '' This caller's comment was sheer nonsense. There are literally hundreds of reasons why baldness takes place and wearing a hat is not one of them.

At least thirty-seven additional types of alopecia could be mentioned, but many of them are so very rare they needn't be defined, unless we come across them in discussing treated patients. For instance, in Chapters Seven and Eight, is the description of the successful prevention and immediate reversal of *alopecia medicamentosa,* diffuse hair loss, most notably from the scalp, caused by the administration of cytotoxic chemotherapy for cancer.

Among the striking anatomical features of human hair are its distribution, its variety, and its sparsity compared with that of other primates. Human hair is not vestigial; it varies in type, density, and length. The hair strands and their follicles have a unique anatomy unlike any other structures in or on the human body. Our next chapter will discuss that uniqueness.

CHAPTER THREE

The Anatomy of Hair and Its Follicles

Despite the technologic revolution we have undergone during the past few decades, the human hair follicle remains a mysterious and intriguing structure. Some of the most basic questions puzzling health care practitioners and their patients about hair growth and hair loss or scalp health and scalp disease remain unanswered. Even with almost all hair follicles being remarkably accessible to observation and study, facts about human hair and scalp physiology continue to seem remote.

Anatomy of the Anagen Hair Follicle

Leonard C. Sperling, M.D., a U.S. Army Major on the Dermatology Service at Walter Reed Army Medical Center in Washington, D.C., points out that hair structure is easily examined through studying clipped hair shafts, entire hairs gently pulled or forcibly plucked from the scalp, and scalp biopsies. These are the means by which anatomic features in the scalp are noted by histologists, dermatologists, internists, biologists, plastic surgeons, and other interested medical/technical professionals. Dr. Sperling writes, "Every day, approximately fifty to one hundred hairs from various regions of the scalp are shed and replaced by newly growing

anagen hair. Anagen follicles are highly active metaboli-
cally, which explains their sensitivity to nutritional deprivation and chemical insult. The vast majority of hairs on the
normal scalp represent anagen follicles."[1]

The term *Anagen*, as used by Dr. Sperling and other
dermatologists, refers to the growing phase of a human hair
strand, and this phase may last at least two years and perhaps
up to five. People with hair colored black, brown, or black/
brown, have 100,000 follicles present in the scalp. Blonds
have about 10 percent more follicles and redheads 10 percent
fewer. Typically, about 90 percent of the hairs are growing
and the balance remain resting or shedding.

With each person possessing somewhere between 90,000
and 120,000 hairs on the head during youth, one can expect
that as many as one hundred hairs a day will let go and fall
onto the pillow, float down the shower drain, or be caught
by a comb or hairbrush. Such shedding is perfectly natural
and presents no cause for alarm. If left uncut during the
anagen phase, hair can grow to forty inches or more.[2] (See
text and diagrams in Chapter Four.)

The anagen growth stage for hair follicles is subdivided
into six substages, the first five of which are collectively
called *proanagen* and are defined by progressively higher
levels of new hair tip position within the follicle; the sixth
stage, *metanagen* is demarcated by emergence of the hair
shaft above the skin surface. When a hair can be seen protrud-
ing from the skin, most often its hair follicle is in the phase
of metanagen.

A useful way to conceptualize the internal organization
of the hair follicle is as a series of concentric cellular compartments. Starting near the bottom, we see that the follicle
is bounded by an acellular *basement membrane* (also referred
to by histologists as a "glassy membrane"). The *outer root
sheath* is the most peripheral of the cellular compartments.
Next comes the *inner root sheath,* which is composed of
three compartments: *Henle's layer, Huxley's layer,* and a
cuticle that forms the bulk of the hair shaft, and the variable
central *medulla.*

The longitudinal organization of the follicle is divided

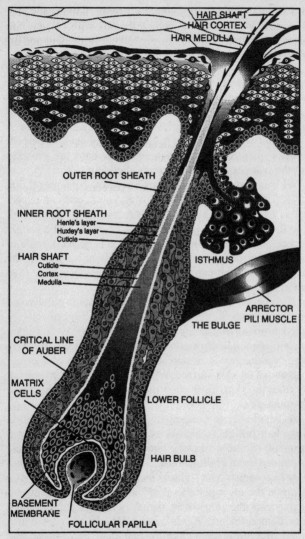

HAIR SHAFT
HAIR CORTEX
HAIR MEDULLA

OUTER ROOT SHEATH

INNER ROOT SHEATH
  Henle's layer
  Huxley's layer
  Cuticle

HAIR SHAFT
  Cuticle
  Cortex
  Medulla

ISTHMUS

ARRECTOR
PILI MUSCLE

THE BULGE

CRITICAL LINE
OF AUBER

MATRIX
CELLS

LOWER FOLLICLE

HAIR BULB

BASEMENT
MEMBRANE

FOLLICULAR PAPILLA

Drawing 3–1 depicts the anatomy of a hair follicle in the metanagen phase. This active growth stage, during which hair is produced and grows toward the outside to protrude above the skin, offers a variety of structures.

into seven regions with distinct anatomic boundaries. The *permanent portion* of the follicle begins with (1) the *hair canal* region, only distinct during fetal development and not present in a person after entry in to the world. It forms the foundation for an actual hair follicle. This hair canal extends from the skin surface to the level of the skin at the epidermal-dermal junction. Its lower part later becomes the intraepidermal "infundibular unit," which comprises the top portion of a follicle.

(2) The *infundibulum* extends down to the level of the opening of the sebaceous duct.

(3) Next is the *area of the sebaceous gland.*

(4) The *isthmus* begins at the sebaceous duct and ends below at the area of the bulge.

(5) The *area of the bulge* is the site of insertion of the arrector pili muscle which causes a hair strand to stand upright. The *transient portion* of the follicle begins at this level and extends to the deepest levels of a follicle.

(6) The *lower follicle* includes the *keratogenous zone* and extends from the area of the bulge to the top of the hair bulb.

(7) The *hair bulb* is the deepest portion of the follicle structure and envelops the follicular papilla. The *critical line of Auber* lies at the widest diameter of the bulb and is of significance in that the bulk of the mitotic activity that gives rise to the hair and inner root sheath occurs below this level.

The hair follicle lies at an angle relative to the skin surface, and the follicle side that forms an acute angle with the skin is its *anterior* aspect; the side that forms an oblique angle is the *posterior.* When the arrector pili muscle contracts, such as in response to cold external temperatures, this tiny muscle pulls on the posterior side and makes the hair stand up as "goose bumps". This associated architectural change in the skin provides a greater thermal barrier as the relative thickness of the insulating medium is increased.

The Hair Follicle Factories

Follicles are the anatomic "factories" that have as their principal function production of the biologic fibers known as hair. These follicles are not static but rather show themselves as dynamic growing, shrinking, and metabolizing structures. They cycle periodically through an "on" state, when hair is produced, and an "off" state, when there is minimal metabolic activity.[3]

The ultimate pattern of activity within follicles in any given area of the scalp or skin in humans is designated as *mosaic* in that adjacent follicles may be functioning in different stages of the hair cycle. (See Chapter Four.) This mosaic pattern is in contrast to many animals, in which there is a *wave* pattern of follicular activity such that adjacent follicles are nearly synchronized, thus facilitating their defined moulting cycles. Although human fetuses and newborns also initially display a wave pattern in utero and during the early postnatal period, this synchronization is later lost. Waves of hair growth occur before establishment of the mosaic pattern, which is usually present by the end of the first postnatal year.[4,5,6,7]

Growth of head hair is differentiated considerably from individual to individual. Average growth rates are about three-fourths inch per month for head hair and one inch per month for beard hair. Female hair grows at about the same speed as male hair.

A single hair does not grow continuously. Typically it increases in length for a few months to five years or so, remains constant in measurement for a time, and then falls out and is replaced. No constancy of the growth pattern exists. Neither cutting nor leaving hair uncut has any important effect on the growth and replacement of the hair. Therapeutic stimulation of new hair must be directed to increasing the hair's follicular energy and neutralizing one's own white blood cell (autoimmune) attack of the hair follicles. Improving the rate of protein replacement, exciting vasodilation of scalp blood vessels, enhancing nutrition to the hair's tiny secretory cavity, reducing hair root inflammation, and accomplishing other positive metabolic effects are also needed.

"Hair is easily affected by changes in nutrition and general health," says Walter Unger, M.D., a dermatologist teaching at the University of Toronto. "Triggers to hair loss [for women] include going off the Pill, severe emotional stress, bad health or crash diets." In those cases, hair returns to its normal growth cycle in three to six months, as the body regains its equilibrium.

Most women also lose hair after a pregnancy. "During pregnancy, hair is in a growth phase because of the hormonal stimulus," explains dermatologist Zoe Draelos, M.D., of Winston-Salem, North Carolina. "Three to nine months after giving birth, all the follicles go into a resting phase—so you end up losing a lot of hair at once." Eventually, most women's hair returns to its prepregnancy status.[8]

All hair growth starts with follicle formation on the fetal head and skin taking form within a pregnant woman's uterus. Primary hair follicles on the head and skin of most body regions appear about the fourth month of gestation in the developing fetus. As mentioned, there's a kind of mosaic pattern of fetal folliculogenesis (formation of follicles) which are not synchronized and show as a randomized onset of follicle formation. The growing anagen follicle appears first and produces a hair. The lanugo (fetal) hairs form on the unborn's body. In the newborn, rougher and coarser terminal hairs make their appearance in the anagen phase. Scalp hairs grow much longer and thicker than the hairs in other body regions during fetal as well as postnatal life. Scalp hair follicles have a more lasting anagen phase than the follicles in other body regions.

Deep in the scalp, the papilla skin cells are responsible for ordering other skin cells to grow hair. If not dead altogether, a bald person's hair follicles may continue to produce hair, only the hair produced is almost invisible, like peach fuzz. If the follicles are damaged but do possess any life at all, with effort and patience they can be stimulated into activity by application of thymus gland extract, a product about which I'll discuss in later chapters.

Listed in **Table 3-1** are some significant characteristics of usual hair growing from the normal average adult human scalp.

TABLE 3–1

Usual Characteristics of Hair Growth on the Body and Scalp[9,10,11,12] (modified from the original medical texts)

- Total body hair follicles on average is an estimated 5 million
- Average number of scalp hairs on someone's head is 100,000
- Age of the fastest hair growth is between 15 and 30 years old
- Slowest growth for hair occurs in infants and the elderly
- Follicular density at birth is 1135 per square centimeter (cm^2)

> at 1 year is 795 per cm^2
> at 15 years is 615 per cm^2
> at 30 years+ is 485 per cm^2
> at 80 years is 435 per cm^2

- Speed of hair growth in the average scalp is 0.35 to 0.44 mm per day
- Speed of hair growth on the body and beard is 0.27 mm per day
- Hair grows faster in summer than in winter for everyone
- Average anagen phase growth cycle is 2 to 5 years
- Average daily loss of hair is 25 to 100 hairs per day
- Female hair grows faster than male hair
- Diameter and shape of hair both vary with a person's race and hair type
- The average age when a man might expect to experience hair loss is between the ages of thirty-five and forty, although many in their twenties start balding.

The Glycosaminoglycan Factor in Hair Growth

The glycosaminoglycan nutrients—natural body components surrounding the perifollicular tissue—have a major influence on hair growth. The glycosaminoglycans are secreted by the perifollicular fibroblasts which are widely distributed cells in connective tissue. Such fibroblasts are responsible for the production of collagen, elastic fibers, and reticular fibers in the skin, and they increase with age of the individual.

The glycosaminoglycans are primarily deposited in the skin papillae, which are one of the growth centers of the hair follicle. They can be altered, regulated, or deregulated by a variety of adverse circumstances affecting the scalp such as starvation, generalized malnutrition, nutritional deficiency, toxic metal syndrome, environmental pollution, emotional stress, autoimmune disease, metabolic disorders, blocked oil glands, dirt embedded into the skin, disruption of the proteoglycan biosynthesis, aging, or androgenetic hormones. The skin of the scalp and the hair that evolves from that scalp reflects the body's overall condition.[13,14]

Advertised hair-growing items and therapies which fail to take into account immunological function, oily gland blockage with sebum, hair follicle metabolism, and the other factors mentioned above cannot possibly work to restore hair.[15]

The Internal Structure of a Hair Strand

Many differentiations exist in the internal structure of a hair strand. For example, the individual hair's central medulla variably may be continuous and pigment-filled, continuous and empty, discontinuous, broken, or fragmented. The thickness of the hair's outer layer, referred to as *the cortex,* and the amount and size of the pigment granules also differ considerably. The *cuticle,* or outer layer of the hair, is covered by a multitude of fine, scale-like markings which represent the attachment of the root sheath during growth in the follicle. These markings on hair are highly characterisitic of the individual, and thus utilized in identification. There is even more variation, however, in the hundreds of thousands of hairs on one person's head, and a single hair (or a few strands) may not be typical of the individual. Unlike a fingerprint, therefore, a hair strand does not provide a precise means of identifying someone.[16]

Hair consists chemically of a highly insoluble substance, the protein-like keratin, containing a fixed proportion of the amino acids arginine, histidine, and lycine but variable proportions of cystine. Keratin, a usual component of skin, reaches its highest concentration of 15 percent in human hair. Sebaceous glands opening about the neck of the hair follicle provide a natural, protective, oily covering, which is further distributed by brushing and grooming.[17]

Hair is a cylinder of impacted keratinized cells comprising three major structures: the outside layer called the *cuticle,* the next layer labeled the cortex, and the central-most layer known as the *medulla* (see **Drawing 3-2**).

The *medulla* contains melanin pigment granules and is present only in thick terminal hair. It is the least important part of the hair as pertains to a hair product which nourishes or stimulates hair regrowth.[18]

The *cortex,* the thickened part of the hair shaft, is a site at which most of the hair's changes of texture, porosity, brittleness, color and thickness occurs.[19]

The *cuticle,* consisting of flattened cells arranged like shingles on a roof, maintains the integrity of the hair shaft. The overlapping is extremely tight, preventing damage to the underlying cortex. The scale-like cells overlap in a proximal-to-distal direction (from the hair's origin to its end) along the hair shaft. When the cuticle is intact, the scales are smooth, refect light, and provide the hair with a shiny, healthy look. This healthy appearance is a manifestation of the hair's porosity, elasticity, and texture.

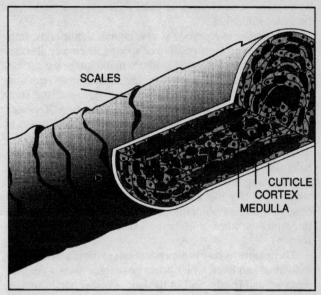

Drawing 3–2 Shows the anatomy of a typical hair shaft with its medulla and cortex, plus the cuticle that is formed by shingle-like scales.

Porous, Elastic, and Textured Hair Health

The porosity of a hair is its ability to absorb moisture, which in good hair health allows only a minimal amount of water or other substances to penetrate through the cuticle into the cortex. When permanent wave or color reactions take place in the cortex, they do so because the cuticle has been rendered vulnerable or open. By increasing the temperature or by changing the pH of the environment around the shaft, the scales of the cuticle are separated and chemicals are allowed inside the cortex. These cuticular scales gradually close again when the processing of hair is finished. If the hair is processed too many times, the cuticle never quite returns to its original tightness and the barrier becomes imperfect.

Hair that is overporous is dry, contains split ends, fractures easily, and feels gummy or spongy when wet. Besides chemical processing, other methods that damage the cuticle, such as blow-drying, wind, sun, and curling irons, can also affect porosity. If the cuticle becomes damaged, the shaft swells with water whenever the hair is washed. Repeated expansion and contraction of the hair shaft gradually weakens it.

The elasticity, or the measure of the tensile strength of hair, allows a healthy hair shaft to stretch to 1.33 times its original length when wet and return to its original length when dry.[20] Dry hair can usually support the stretch or pull of a 100-gram weight without breaking. Hair passes through three phases when it is being extended under increasing force.[21]

The texture of hair is dependent on (a) the diameter of the individual hair fiber, which affects its degree of coarseness or fineness, and (b) the feel of the hair, whether harsh, soft, or wiry.

The hair's permeability, how easily fluids or gases flow through the shafts and pedicles of hair into their follicles, is affected by the three major characteristics of a hair shaft—porosity, elasticity, and texture. If hair follicles continue to be alive even in an area of bare scalp, and the dormant hair follicles could give rise to hair shafts with good permeability, chances are that the application of a well-recommended nourishing/stimulating hair treatment and shampoo will stimulate new or revitalized hair growth.

A Body Clock that Controls the Hair Growth Cycle

What is the nature of a person's internal "clock" which controls the hair growth cycle and where in the follicle is it situated? As yet, plastic surgeons and dermatologists cannot answer such intriguing questions. While recent years have seen a number of advances in hair biology, tissue interactions which include androgen-regulating responses, leucocytic immune attacks on follicles, and hair pigmentation loss remain unknown.[22]

A few of the world's medical specialists offering hair treatment are beginning to understand the molecular basis of hair growth control, although the picture is still far from clear for them too. This is the reason that the manner of action of a hair regrowth product remains uncertain even among its clinical exponents. Observing its excellence in reversing the incidence of hair loss for numerous patients, they know that calf thymus extract works but not entirely why. There are educated conjectures based on the evidence, of course, but they come down to being mere theories based on principles.

In the following chapter, we will see that hair follicles periodically cycle between growth and resting stages, and there are various types of hair which are classified according to their texture and length.[23]

CHAPTER FOUR

Growth Stages of Hair and Their Problems

In the heart of London, at the hair clinic of a second-floor walk-up off Leicester Square, middle-aged and motherly Cockney clerks dispense thick tubes of tars, creams or ointments, apply stinky potions, and occasionally attach terrifying contraptions to the heads of people with falling or absent hair. One of the more peculiar items is an electrical device crackling with static that looks like it should be strapped to the head of Frankenstein's monster. What these ingredients and machines are supposedly doing is awakening hair follicles into a spurt of hair strand growth. If the hair follicles have any life to them at all, there's a chance that these variable ingredients may do something to stimulate follicular growth.

As previously explained, hair follicles are the biologic "factories" within which production of the hair shafts or strands are accomplished. The major physiological purposes of body and head hair for most mammals are: the conservation of body heat, the offering of camouflage, and as a means of generalized external and internal protection. (In particular, ear hairs and nasal hairs serve this protective purpose.) In modern humans, hair has also become a means of social organization, of sexual signaling, and a factor in appropriate appearance. Thus, hair on the head and body has multiple purposes for use by the human organism. It arises in a unique fashion starting within the mother's uterus at that stage when an embryo begins to turn into a fetus.

Three Types of Human Hair

The embryonic cells which eventually develop into a hair follicle are first evident in the human fetus at about the eighth or ninth week of pregnancy. They are distributed mainly in the areas of the eyebrows, upper lip, and chin. Most of the remaining follicles begin to ripen at approximately four to five months' gestation in a direction either toward the head (cephalad) or toward the tail bone (caudad) and not out to the sides of a fetus' developing body.

The production of these newly spreading follicles occurs in several interspersed waves producing typical groupings of three hairs. (Please refer to **Drawing 3-1** in the previous chapter.) *Matrix cells,* located above the *basement membrane* overlying the skin's *follicular papilla,* give rise to the *hair shaft* and the *inner root sheath. Melanocytes* responsible for the pigmentation of the hair are dispersed among these matrix cells. Development of the associated *sebaceous gland* and *arrector pili muscle* completes the major structures of the entire *pilosebaceous apparatus* of the hair follicle.[1]

The first type of hair that appears on an individual at birth is called *lanugo* hair. It is non-pigmented, very fine, and wispy. When one sees a newborn who has thick, dark head hair it's an indication that the mother's hormonal influences on the fetus provided strong stimuli for such growth. This hair falls out after birth because the mother ceases to feed the fetus through its placenta.

Lanugo hairs get shed and replaced by either *vellus* or *terminal* hairs. Vellus hair, the fine, tiny nonpigmented hair strands covering most of the body, feels soft and velvety.

Terminal hair is more crude or coarse such as the type that grows across the head, under the arms, in the pubic region, or on the chest, legs, and arms. Terminal hair is strong, long, colored, and amounts to somewhere around 100,000 to 120,000 strands growing from the scalp. (Estimates of how much hair grows on a person's head varies from one authority to the next, fluctuating from 90,000 strands to 150,000.) A person at twenty years of age will likely have his or her thickest head of hair. During the mid-twenties, hair quantity begins to decrease and continues to disminish at a regular rate—fast or slow, depending on sex and hereditary traits—until death. As one gets older, the head hair grows thinner (see **Table 3-1** in the previous chapter and **Table 4-1** later in this chapter).

When a terminal strand of hair is in its first stage and growing, dermatologists designate the head and body hair as being in its *anagen phase.* The Greek word *ana* means "going up" or "over," and the Greek word *gen* indicates "growth" or "life." Hence, an *anagen* hair is one that is growing up or full of life. This anagen phase for a single terminal hair lasts from twenty-four to sixty months, averaging four years. It progresses in growth at the rate of three-fourths inch per month; therefore, in forty-eight months, a single hair if left uncut and not broken could theoretically grow to be three feet long or longer.

A second stage in the hair strand's growth cycle is the *catagen* phase. From the Greek, *cata* relates to "going down," so the catagen phase is a state of suspended animation of hair with no growth, a sleeping stage that lasts for approximately fourteen to twenty-eight days. During this period, the blood supply slows to the hair root and slowly shuts off. The hair root shrinks, and cells in the papilla (tiny areas at the hair base that provide blood for hair growth) slowly stop dividing.

The final stage of a strand's growth cycle, lasting for up to but never more than five months, is the *telogen phase,* with *tel* from the Greek meaning "the end". Hence, a hair in the telogen phase is at the end of its growth. It possesses a superficial root which allows it to be pulled out easily when combs and brushes are run through the hair. If not combed out, eventually the telogen hair gets forced out by a new hair growing from the same follicle. The new arrival has entered its own anagen phase.[2] (See **Drawing 4-1.**)

Hairs are released from the scalp normally at the rate of

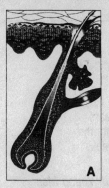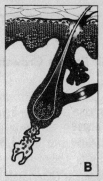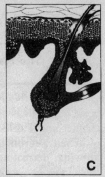

Drawing 4–1 is a medical illustrator's rendition showing the three phases of the hair growth cycle.

(A) The mid-growth anagen phase in which the hair shaft is firmly embedded and a hair strand is growing.

(B) The mid-growth catagen phase in which a club structure has formed as the outer hair root sheath collapses and withdraws up the follicular sheath. The hair is sleeping.

(C) The ending telogen phase in which the follicle is shrinking as the sheath retracts and trails in the dermal layer of the scalp below. Here, the hair strand is getting ready to let go and fall out in the normal cycle of hair growth.

approximately eighty strands daily, and get replaced from underneath. Each hair strand has its own timetable, some in phases of anagen, others in catagen (or catatonic phase), and additional ones become telogen when they are about to let go. Unlike some animals such as elk and reindeer, humans don't shed massive quantities of hair in a growth cycle.[3]

Table 4–1 and **Table 4–2** offer a summary of information about hair follicles, their growth cycles, and the hair strands that arise from them.

TABLE 4–1

The Hair Follicle Growth Cycle[4,5]

In the Adult Scalp Three Growth Phases Exist

Anagen phase	2–5 years
Telogen phase	2–5 months
Catagen phase	2–4 weeks

Length of Anagen at Other Sites in Young Men

Legs	5–7 months
Arms	1.5–3 months
Fingers	1–3 months
Eyelashes	1–6 months

Normal Adult Scalp Hair Loss Is 50 to 100 hairs per day

TABLE 4–2

Hair Follicle Statistical Data[6]

Number of adult anagen hair follicles present	80%–85%–90%
Number of adult telogen hair follicles present	10%–15%–18%
Number of child anagen hair follicles present	95%
Number of child telogen hair follicles present	5%
Mean adult scalp hair shaft diameter	70 microns

Testing for Anagen Effluvium as a Cause of Baldness

Inasmuch as the hair of monkeys and other primates is a great deal like human hair, much research on hair growth and loss is in experiments performed on them. Hideo Uno, M.D., Ph.D., Senior Scientist at the Wisconsin Regional Primate Research Center and Adjunct Associate Professor in the Department of Pathology and Laboratory Medicine at the University of Wisconsin in Madison, states: "In structure and function the anagen follicle is virtually an independent factory that manufactures hair, maintains its own sheath, and stores the basic energy supply. Hair loss occurs in many pathophysiological conditions of the skin as well as in systemic disorders. Classification of hair loss is commonly divided into two categories, cicatricial (scarring) and noncicatricial alopecia.

"Noncicatricial alopecia is caused by either functional or structural disorders of the hair follicle itself. This latter condition may be further divided into primary and secondary causes. Secondary follicular disorders are usually the result of chemotherapy or physical (radiation) treatments of cancers, nutritional and hormonal disorders, or stress," says Dr. Uno. "Although the cause and pathogenetic backgrounds of primary noncicatricial alopecia are largely unknown, this refractory and mostly irreversible hair loss has been a major therapeutic challenge for the dermatologists."[7]

An acute, extreme alteration of growth of the majority of anagen follicles known as *anagen effluvium* results in acute loss of greater than 85 percent of the scalp hair (considerable baldness). There is a simple way to corroborate that abnormal hair loss is coming from anagen effluvium-by a *hair pull* test. It's a main diagnostic tool used by dermatologists and quite easy for anyone who suspects a problem to try.

Here is how a hair pull test is done: Simply grasp the base of a clump of fifty to one hundred hairs between thumb and forefinger and gently pull on the hair proximally to distally (from the scalp outward). Normally only a total of two to five telogen hairs will be obtained in this manner, depending on how recently the hair was shampooed and styled. Shampooing will have removed most of the readily shed telogen hairs. The longer the period since shampooing, the more telogen hairs will be obtained in a hair pull. Do this hair pull test seven times, and if twelve to twenty hairs come away on average each time, there is a diagnosable scalp disorder. It comes from anagen effluvium—an acknowledged pathological condition.

To confirm any suspicions, collect in plastic bags a week's span of hairs gotten from the hair pull test. Also collect all hairs shed in the shower, sink, brush, and on the counter, pillow, etc. Count and average all hairs in the bags. Remember, the daily normal loss is supposed to be from fifty to one hundred hairs per day at the maximum.[8,9]

Admittedly counting hairs is tedious, but the test is necessary to make a determination as to whether the hair loss is abnormal anagen effluvium or a less abnormal condition of telogen effluvium.

Anagen effluvium merely refers to the abnormal loss of hair during the anagen phase, often seen following administration of certain cancer chemotherapeutic agents. It also comes from exposure to some chemicals or it can arrive in association with various other factors and diseases.

Telogen effluvium is different. It's the early, excessive, temporary loss of normal club hairs from normal resting follicles in the scalp. It arises as a result of traumatization by some stimulus such as surgery, starvation diet, parturition, drugs, traction on the hair (as with braiding), high fever, certain diseases, psychogenic stress or other sources shown in Table 4–3 that follows. Therefore telogen effluvium is an altering of the normal hair cycle which may prematurely precipitate the anagen phase into the catagen and telogen phases.

The hair pull test can be used as a simple, easily-applied

tool to follow the progress of one's own hair loss or regrowth. **Table 4-3** contains a diagnostic differential of the many reasons for hair loss.

TABLE 4–3[10,11]

Differential Diagnosis of Hair Loss

Nonscarring Hair Loss

Diffuse hair loss
Hair breakage
Anagen effluvium
Mercury poisoning from dental amalgams
Thallium poisoning
Hair shaft disorder
Physical stress
Chemical poisoning
Telogen effluvium
Childbirth
Fever episodes
Surgery
Drug use
Excessive androgens
Nutritional metabolic disorders
Autoimmune disease
Chronic scalp disease
Androgenetic alopecia in women
Alopecia totalis or universalis
Loose anagen syndrome
Failure of or abnormal production of hormones

Focal (local) cause of hair loss
Infection
Traumatic
Alopecia areata

    Hair breakage
    Androgenic alopecia in men and women
    Development

Scarring Hair Loss

    Inflammatory hair loss
       Lupus erythematosus
       Lichen planus pilaris
       Planopilaris
       Pseudopelade
       Scleroderma
       Bullous pemphigoid
       Epidermolysis bullosa acquista
       Folliculitis—secondary to infectious agents
       Chemical and physical damage
       Granulomatous inflammation

    Noninflammatory hair loss
       Nonscarring pseudopelade
       Bullous pemphigoid
       Neoplasms
          Benign
          Malignant

The Diagnosis of Alopecia Areata

Alopecia areata is classified as one of the focal conditions associated with telogen effluvium. Dermatologists and other hair specialists must distinguish a cause from the various reasons for hair loss. The reasons for alopecia areata include male/female pattern baldness from excessive androgens in men and/or women, allergies, abuse of street drugs, adverse side effects to prescription medications, nutritional deficiencies, pesticides and herbicides, toxic metals such as mercury amalgam materials used for dental fillings, immune suppression from latent infections under dental root canals, the many over-the-counter drugs, alcoholic beverages, excessive traction by braiding hair too tightly, fungal infections, hair dyes, cancers and moles, thyroid disease, familial traits, genetic tendencies, and more.

The complexity of baldness turns out to be a syndrome, a group of signs and symptoms that occur together and are typical of the particular disorder. For instance, when bald spots develop rather suddenly within a few weeks, these are telltale signs of alopecia universalis, a relatively common form of alopecia areata. The condition appears as one or more smooth, unscarred, completely hairless round or oval patches on the scalp. It's totally unlike the gradual loss of hair in common balding.

The perplexing syndrome of sudden baldness, therefore, could encompass all the hair on a person's body, including the eyelashes and eyebrows. The more extensive the loss, the less likely it is that any known treatment will prompt the hair to regrow, even though the affected hair follicles remain alive and potentially able to function again normally. The immune system, gone awry from some of the antigens with which people are in contact daily, is suspected of being the source of this universal hair loss. (An antigen is a foreign substance in the body to which it responds by forming an antibody.) Antigens cause adverse allergic reactions—probably including hair loss.

Medical science is hardly able to furnish good answers to some penetrating questions about baldness, but what some doctors I've interviewed believe is that alopecia areata behaves like an autoimmune disease in which the body's immune system attacks its own tissues. The target of this immune attack seems to be the hair follicles. When examined under a microscope, the dormant follicles are typically surrounded by lymphocytes, macrophages, and other white blood cells produced when the body sets off an immunological response to an offending agent like infectious bacteria—one of the types of antigens.

Still, if a bald person could uncover the antigen or deficiency, toxicity, drug-relationship, radiation, dental root canal or other source of alopecia universalis and get rid of the underlying pathology, that person could regrow hair on the head and body by the faithful application of *Thymu-Skin®* Shampoo and Hair Treatment lotion. I make this statement with the assurance that alopecia universalis has been reversed numerous times already with the use of this calf thymus preparation, one of the many therapies being discussed in this book. Clinical investigations in Germany and Austria, some of them using the scientific method of random-selection, placebo-control, and double-blind, are the proof that specific hair loss problems such as among the anagen hair shedding (effluvium) of the alopecias can be corrected permanently.[12]

Since up to 90 percent of scalp hair may be in anagen at any given time, anagen hair loss is more extensive. For reasons not yet determined, dermatologists more commonly are consulted by people exhibiting telogen shedding. The only way that a dermatologist is able to tell if the patient has anagen or telogen effluvium is to look at the hair strands under the microscope to recognize their distinct hair shaft characteristics.

German medical professors and other clinicians report that women of all ages respond well—more readily than men—to the topical application of the calf thymus extract for either anagen or telogen hair loss when no permanent scarring alopecia has taken place.

CHAPTER FIVE

Why Some Women Lose Their Hair or See It Grow Thin

History's most famous fairy tale about a "damsel-in-distress" tells how Rapunsel used her head by lowering her long tresses to aid in her rescue from the tower prison. But just suppose the lovely lady had loose-rooted hair strands like so many women of today. Might she have remained in the tower, and bald-headed at that? If even the slightest bit fragile or thinning, her hair could have been a tragic let-down . . . .

When it comes to the fairer sex, nothing is more unfair than hair loss. While about 66 percent of all adult males in Western industrialized countries experience some form of thinning hair and 40 percent of them actually develop observable baldness, women are not too far behind. According to The National Alopecia Areata Foundation in both the United States and Canada, nearly 22 percent of all the world's women will experience various types of hair loss during their lives.

The Root of Her Hair Loss

Look at the case of Elline Surianello, who told her sad story in the February 1992 issue of the *Ladies Home Journal*. At the young age of twenty-nine, she was going bald. Her hairline was deeply receding, and the hair on the top of Elline's head was so scant one could see scalp shining through the thin strands It's true that most people consider baldness a man's problem. Yet an estimated twenty million American women—nearly one of every five—suffer some degree of hair loss, from thinning hair and patchy bald spots to no body hair at all.[1]

For females, abnormal hair loss can come from a wide assortment of causes. Androgenetic alopecia in women, also known as female-patterned baldness, is a sure sign that the body is in distress. The well-known feminist physician who is a Fellow of the American College of Obstetricians and Gynecologists, Christiane Northrup, M.D., said in an interview, "The body often gets the message before the brain. . . . No symptom is purely physical or purely psychological."[2]

Commenting on the known reasons for a woman to go bald, Elline Surianello advised her readers that some hair loss can be traced to hormonal changes or medical problems. But the most common cause for women is a hereditary condition known as androgenetic alopecia, or female pattern baldness. All of Elline's aunts on her father's side were balding and wore scarves or topknots to cover their thinning hair. But the stigma of her own baldness was so great that friends and family never dared to acknowledge the problem. "Your hair looks all right," people would tell her. Out of an act of kindness, they were lying, of course.

Elline reveals that even as a small child, her hair was very sparse; her mother used to shave the child's head in a futile attempt to make Elline's hair grow thicker. As she grew older, the girl tried everything—pills, potions, tonics, shampoos that promised to make her hair thicker. In sadness, she states that nothing worked. Dermatologists and nutritionists could do nothing. "You just have thin hair," they'd say.

The hormonal changes of puberty only made her hair loss worse. While all of Elline's friends were working at department stores or fast-food restaurants, she took a job in a wig shop and spent her paychecks buying wigs in every length, color and style. People thought she was having fun with her crazy hairpieces. No one knew how much Elline loathed them. She hated them most during the summer months, when her scalp would perspire and itch. She worried constantly that the fake hair was crooked or that a strong wind would blow it off. The young woman didn't date because she couldn't bear the thought of being with a boy and having her wig come off. Elline didn't even go to her senior prom.

Finally, Elline Surianello stopped wearing wigs when she was nineteen. Why? Because she hated the way even a good wig made her appear in public, and she tried to ignore the problem the same way a woman might ignore a run in her stockings, hoping no one will notice. She wore flashy jewelry and eccentric clothes to detract attention from the looks of her hair. After earning her business degree, Elline left the wig shop and accepted a job in a cosmetics company where she works today. In fact, Elline Surianello never did find any permanent solution for her hair loss. Even now, she just suffers with her typical pattern of androgenetic alopecia.

The Common Baldness of Androgenetic Alopecia

Common baldness, known medically as *androgenetic alopecia,* results from the double combination: (a) too adequate a supply of natural androgen from one's endocrine system, and (b) the appropriate genetic background acquired from parents and family. A more correct spelling of the medical term for common baldness might be *andro-genetic alopecia* to emphasize both requisite factors: androgens and a genetic predisposition.[3]

Both men and women may be affected by this process of alopecia but the patterns of hair loss are usually quite distinct for the two sexes. For male/female pattern baldness comparisons, see **Drawing 5-1** and **Drawing 5-2.**

There are differences in common baldness patterns among men and women. For men, the eight typical patterns of andro-genetic alopecia (Grades I, II, III, IIIvertex, IV, V, VI, and VII) were arrived at by the American dermatologist John B. Hamilton, M.D., in 1951.[4] For women, the three typical patterns of andro-genetic alopecia (Grades I, II, and III) were developed by British dermatologist Edward Ludwig, M.D., in 1977.[5]

As determined by dermatologist Klio Moessler, M.D., of the Darmstadt Municipal Clinics in Darmstadt, Germany, and Professor Manfred Hagedorn, M.D., Chief of the Dermatology Department at the University of Frankfurt in Darmstadt, this androgenetic alopecia problem has responded for no less than 99 percent of Germany's bald women when *Thymu-Skin®* was applied by them faithfully.

Active shedding of hair from andro-genetic alopecia, as well as with many other types of hair shedding, is not uncommonly associated with scalp discomfort or tenderness upon hair manipulation. Some alopecia patients feel low grade pain in the scalp at the root of their hair strands.

Androgenetic alopecia for some women results from transformation of terminal hair follicles to vellus-like hair follicles, which in the later stages become atrophic. They waste away from normal development due to spontaneous degeneration of the hair follicle's cells. This may occur through undernourishment, disuse, or aging. My seventeen-year-old granddaughter, Caren Michelle Walker, has a girlfriend who suffers from alopecia directly resulting from her anorexia nervosa. Whole clumps of hair fall from her head and remain behind after she has lounged on a piece of furniture. This happens simply because her hair follicles' cells are malnourished.

Anorexia nervosa is a psychological illness, most common in female adolescents, in which the patients have no desire to eat; eating, in fact, becomes abhorrent to them. The problem often starts with a simple desire to lose weight, which then becomes an obsession. The result is severe loss of weight plus other symptoms such as hair loss. Since the hair follicles' cells subdivide faster than any other body cells, (except perhaps for that of the bone marrow and gastric mucosa), much nourishment is needed. With malnutrition from not eating, the individual suffering from anorexia nervosa will show an acute loss of hair.

The progression of andro-genetic alopecia is gradual for

Male—Pattern Baldness

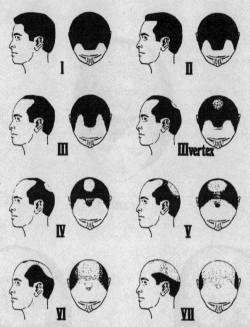

Drawing 5–1 is reproduced from the 1951 *Annals of the New York Academy of Science.* It shows typical common baldness patterns of male andro-genetic alopecia. Seen are (I) the male youngster's normal hair pattern before puberty; (II) the teenager's normal hairline changed at puberty and beginning to recede as the young adult matures; (III) In adulthood, the early stages of baldness occurs, characterized by minimal thinning of hair density and further elevation of the forehead; (IIIvertex) spot balding begins to take place in a patch at the top of the head, the vertex; (IV–VII) progressively more severe patterns of baldness appear until most hair follicles have been damaged or are dead. If follicles have died, no hair regrowth is possible. When they merely lie damaged and dormant, restoration of hair growth is potentially able to be accomplished if an appropriate stimulant is incorporated in the man's daily routine of living. Thymus gland extract, the primary therapeutic ingredient in Thymu-Skin®, is just such a hair-growing stimulant. Clinical tests performed at German Universities indicate that Thymu-Skin® awakens sleeping hair follicles in 67 percent of those men who apply it.

Female—Pattern Baldness

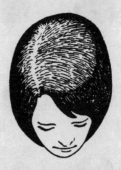

Grade 1

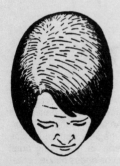

Grade 2

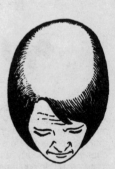

Grade 3

Drawing 5–2 is reproduced from the *British Journal of Dermatology*. This artist's rendition depicts the typical patterns of andro-genetic alopecia which are characteristic (from left to right) of Grade 1, Grade 2, and Grade 3 female pattern baldness.

most women, but there is a steady advance over time of female pattern baldness from its Grades 1 and 2, into 3. This progression happens because successive follicular cycles produce hairs of shorter lengths and decreased diameters.

Endocrinologically normal women with andro-genetic alopecia more often, but not always, exhibit a diffuse hair loss (see **Drawing 5-2**). The process may become apparent at any time after puberty in either sex. If the problem is manifest in a young woman, endocrinologic evaluation by laboratory testing should be considered. Such evaluation is especially indicated if significant acne, hirsuitism (excessive hairiness of the face, arms, and other body parts), or virilization (increased muscle bulk and/or deepening of the voice) are also present. Laboratory testing of this nature is done to determine whether a source of excessive androgens is present.

The Action of Androgens in Hair Loss

In her assessment of the importance of androgens as a source of hair loss, Elline Surianello, cited above, is correct. The steroid hormones known as androgens, exemplified by natural testosterone and other masculine hormones, increase the growth of male physical qualities in men certainly, but in women as well. They are the most important systemic modulators of human hair growth and hair loss in both sexes.

It's known that men castrated before the age of puberty neither grow beards nor go bald unless they are treated with testosterone. Castration of older men prevents the progression of baldness but does not reverse it.

According to Dr. Klio Moessler of the Darmstadt Municipal Clinics, ''Another source of baldness in women may be their own excess of male-type androgens and insufficient quantities of female-type androgens such as estrogen, inasmuch as in androgenic alopecia there is hyperandrogenenia (the presence of excess androgens). For example, in the presence of tumors of the ovaries or the adrenal glands, androgens are produced. In the common baldness of androgenetic alopecia, the patients exhibit normal blood serum androgens. But due to their genetic dispositions, some women with female pattern baldness have hair loss because an enzyme (5-alpha-reductase) gives rise to another hormone that I had discussed previously. It's known chemically as

5-alpha-dihydrotestosterone (5-alpha-DHT) and derives from the body's own testosterone. This hormonal 5-alpha-DHT acts with a receptor that is present within the responsive hair follicle," advises Dr. Moessler.

Pregnancy, Contraception, and Other Reasons for Hair Loss

In the case of hair loss or hair thinning in a woman, there are additional questions about trauma and stress, diet, drugs taken during the prior few months, family history of hair loss, recent illnesses, systemic disease, and other items of note that are specific for the female gender (see **Table 5-1**). For instance, any gynecologist anxious to help a patient suffering with thinning hair likely will ask about her menstrual cycles, pregnancies, abortions, and menopause.

Female hair loss definitely is a gynecological subject as illustrated by some of the studies conducted at the Department of Obstetrics and Gynecology, Division of Gynecological Endocrinology, University of Heidelberg, not only by Drs. Hagedorn and Moessler, but also by the Heidelberg gynecologists T.Rabe, K. Grunwald, L. Kiesel, and B. Runnebaum. Their gynecological studies tied to hair loss and regrowth will be discussed in Chapter Nine.

While pregnant, a woman does not lose as much hair as usual. However, after she delivers her baby, many hairs will enter the resting (catagen) phase of the hair cycle. Within two to three months after delivery, some women will see vast amounts of loose hair being caught in their brushes and combs. This increased shedding lasts between one-to-six months before reversing itself and is recognized in obstetrics as *postpartum telogen effluvium.* It's definitely hormonally based.[6] Not all new mothers experience the hair loss condition, and not all women will notice increased hair thinning with every pregnancy. Still, falling hair is relatively common immediately following childbirth.

Oral contraceptives contain two ingredients which are

significant for head hair: synthetic estrogen and synthetic progesterone (progestin). Women who lose hair while taking birth control pills usually are predisposed to hereditary thinning. Such hair thinning will be hastened by the hormone-like effects common to some of the progestational agents. When a woman stops taking the Pill, she may notice that her hair begins shedding slightly after two to three months. This state is likely to continue for six months, at which time, the situation usually reverses itself spontaneously.[7,8,9]

TABLE 5–1[10]

Summary of Reasons for a Woman's Loss of Hair

Trauma: Physical Injury from a Violent or Disruptive Action
Mental or Emotional Shock and Other Stress
A Poisonous Substance Spreading Through the Body

Pregnancy and Postpartum Reaction

Psychogenic Disorders such as Trichotillomania (the impulse to pull out one's hair)

Infection (Fungal or Bacterial)

Chemical Poisoning

Pharmaceutical Usage: Prescription, Over-the-counter, or Recreational Drug Side Effects

Seborrhea: Excessive Oil Gland Secretions with Associated Facial Lesions

Psoriasis: Inborn Skin Disorder Producing Silvery Scales and Red Patches

Endocrinopathies: Endocrine Gland Dysfunctions

Alopecia Areata: Well-defined Oval or Round, nonscarring Bald Patches

Systemic Illness: Cancer, Lupus Erythematosis, and Other Diseases

Androgenetic Alopecia: Female Pattern Baldness

Age-related: Eventual Hair Loss with Aging

A Case Report of Postpartum Hair Loss

In March 1991, Else L. Heinrich of Frankfurt, Germany, a happily married thirty-two-year-old woman who had undergone one prior miscarriage and subsequent temporary thinning of the hair, gave birth to a healthy baby. But she lost a lot more hair within four weeks of the delivery. Mrs. Heinrich's hair finally stopped falling after a year, but no new growth returned and bare scalp was apparent. Then, the new mother's baldness worsened even further over the next six months after she stopped nursing. Her obstetrician/gynecologist tried many remedies but after another half-year managed to do nothing much to help her. Wearing a wig became a way of life, for she remained totally bald (see **Photograph 5-1**).

Mrs. Heinrich had taken no medications other than oral contraceptives. She complained of feeling tired all the time. Results of the patient's physical examination and history were normal, but her laboratory examination revealed hypothyroidism (a low thyroid level) and infection with Epstein-Barr virus (EBV), causing chronic fatigue syndrome.

These abnormalities—prior pregnancy, discontinuance of nursing, using oral contraceptives, hypothyroidism, EBV infection—could have triggered her underlying androgenetic alopecia, said a skin specialist at the Municipal Clinics at Darmstadt.

Else L. Heinrich eventually got rid of her alopecia within another six months of applying the *Thymu-Skin®* hair treatment program (see **Photograph 5-2**) which is recommended by the entire dermatological staff at the Darmstadt Hospital in Germany.

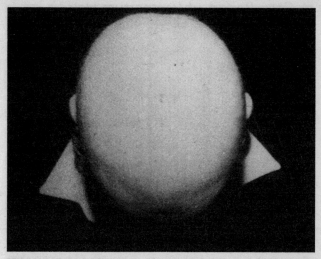

Photograph 5–1 (above) shows the baldness of thirty-two-year-old Else L. Heinrich of Frankfurt, Germany, in April 1992. She suffers from alopecia totalis, a possible result of her dormant androgenetic alopecia triggered by pregnancy or another of the complicating health factors which were affecting her. They included hypothyroidism, discontinuance of nursing six months before, an Epstein-Barr virus infection causing chronic fatigue syndrome, and the use of oral contraceptives.

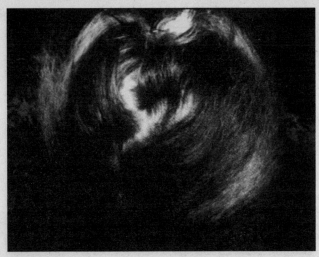

Photograph 5–2 (above) shows new head hair growth on the same woman in November 1992. Else L. Heinrich began the daily application of *Thymu-Skin*® Shampoo and Hair Treatment liquid just one-half year before. Her alopecia totalis is completely gone and hair growth remains normal to this day.

CHAPTER SIX

Chemotherapy as a Cause of Hair Loss

The ingestion of therapeutic drugs and medications has become as commonplace in the industrialized countries of Asia, Australia, North and South America, and Europe as the food people eat, the water they drink, and the air they breathe. Biochemists, physicians, and other scientists through the years, have attempted to increase their understanding of drugs and medications and what effects they can have on us. Depending on amounts ingested, all of them are poisonous—some more than others.

It's not possible even to imagine how much humankind pollutes the planet with commercial chemicals of convenience and industrialization. Not even measuring how much chemical waste is created in other industrialized countries, just consider this: Each year the United States alone produces about 400 billion pounds of synthetic organic chemicals which is equivalent to eighty pounds per year for every single individual living on Earth. Exposure to these American-made toxic chemicals—55,000 in production and 48,000 listed by the Environmental Protection Agency (EPA)-damages our cells.[1] Such chemicals do damage in several ways. They (1) interfere in one or more of the complex biochemical processes that keep one's body going, (2) substitute for a necessary nourishing substance, or (3) adversely affect the body's filters such as the liver, kidneys, lungs, and lymph which help to cleanse our functional physiology.

As explained by nutritional biochemist William Randall Kellas, Ph.D., and Andrea Sharon Dworkin, N.D., Ph.D., in their book, *Surviving the Toxic Crisis,* ''Many things influence the way chemicals affect a particular person. Some chemicals target a particular organ, while other effects are determined by individual genetic 'weak links' in each person—the *genetic translator.* The genetic translator is usually the determinant of symptoms, but some chemicals are so strong that they bypass the genetic translator and go directly to a targeted system.''[2] The cytotoxic agents used for cancer chemotherapy do exactly the latter; they target markedly subdividing cells anywhere in the body. As we will discover in this chapter, hair follicles are most usually among the targeted cells.

The Anagen Alopecia Side Effect of Chemotherapeutic Agents

All chemical poisons may be classified in a variety of ways. The EPA, for example, categorizes them by their:

- *caustic damage* to tissues such as burning and denuding agents,
- *cytotoxicity* (cell poisoning),
- *anoxia* (removal of cellular oxygen),
- *body part effect* on the heart, lungs, liver, kidneys,
- *location* as found in the household, automobiles, medicine cabinet, outdoors, industry,
- *method of ingestion* as through inhalation, swallowing, the skin,
- *application* or use or type exemplified by insecticides, rodenticides, fungicides, herbicides, repellents, paints, solvents,
- *chemical class* as elements, salts, aromatics, halogenated hydrocarbons such as chloroform, chemotherapeutic agents.

For the last item listed, the intent in using chemotherapeutic agents—all of which are toxic, even properly prescribed—is to reduce or eliminate an undesired condition of illness or injury. Doctors are aware, particularly in the case of cytotoxics (cellular poisons) utilized in cancer therapy, that frequently unwanted and unpleasant side effects show up. Too often these adverse side effects themselves cause discomforts, dysfunctions, illnesses, immune suppression, or death.[3]

One important undesirable side effect is the loss of hair (alopecia) during the anagen stage of hair growth. Fortunately anogen alopecia usually reverses itself when the cytotoxic agent is discontinued from therapeutic use. Anticancer drugs and radiation standardly bring about hair fallout within one to three weeks from high doses being administered to patients. Baldness is the consequence, and it represents a serious emotional setback if not a recognized suppressor of the cancer patient's immune system.[4]

At Duke University Medical Center in Durham, North Carolina, oncologist Atif M. Hussein, M.D., confirms in a clinical journal article: ''Alopecia (hair loss) is one of the most physically and psychologically distressing side effects of cancer chemotherapeutic drugs. . . . The threat of anagen alopecia can cause some patients to refuse potentially curative or medically proven adjunctive chemotherapy. Prevention or elimination of this side effect would enhance patient compliance to chemotherapy.''[5]

In an October 20, 1994 interview with one of Germany's leading oncology surgeons, Prof. Dr. med. Ulrich Fink, Chief of the Department of Surgery at the Surgical Clinic and Polyclinic of Technology, the University of Munich, he affirmed that hair loss for his cancer patients invariably was psychologically depressing to their immunological responses. It's an adverse effect matched with nausea and vomiting as the prime source of discomfort for Dr. Fink's patients. He welcomed the legitimate means of saving them from hair loss and does utilize the same anti-alopecia hair treatment program discussed in later chapters. The following chapter, describes how German oncology clinics save their patients from experiencing hair loss which might ordinarily occur from the mandatory prescribing of cytotoxic chemicals.

Chemotherapy Creates More Damage than Hair Loss

Bear in mind that chemotherapeutic agents not only produce a noticeable alopecia effect on the head and body hair but they also bring about an unnoticeable but more life-threatening suppressive effect on the internal organs—the liver, kidneys, heart, blood vessels, and immune system.

In *liver damage,* cancer chemotherapies are responsible for toxic hepatitis, a liver injury with accompanying jaundice resulting in liver cell death (necrosis), and fatty liver. With fatty liver, one cannot process fats and oils properly, so they build up in the arteries and liver to cause high blood pressure (hypertension). Additionally, a situation of dry liver develops. This is a condition in which fat-soluble vitamins A, D, E, and K are not processed for use by the body. Its manifestation is by deficiency symptoms and free radical damage due to loss of the antioxidant effects of vitamins A and E. Dry liver may be compared to a car engine that is allowed to run with insufficient oil. Sooner or later the engine is going to seize up. Both conditions are prevented or remedied by the ingestion of healthy emulsified oils. In addition, the human body responds to an input of choline and lecithin.

In *kidney damage* (renal impairment) resulting from chemotherapy for cancer, there will be altered blood pressure and blood volume, hormonal changes, neurological symptoms, and other systemic effects related to lowered potassium levels. Sugar will show in the urine, urination increases, kidney failure sets in, and ultimately death takes over.

In *heart and blood vessel damage* (cardiovasculitis) from cytotoxicity, hardening of the arteries (atherosclerosis) and hypertension appear. Metallic molecules that make up part of the structure of a chemotherapeutic agent will be deposited in blood vessels as atherosclerotic plaque. Inflammation promoting the release of calcium and cholesterol, gets laid down to buffer the inflammation. From these pathologies come the additional formation of calcium-cholesterol plaque that completely blocks the blood vessels in which it's deposited.

In *immune system damage* from the free radical attack of the cytotoxics, three pathological processes develop. They consist of (a) hypersensitivity with allergy, (b) immune activation leading to autoimmune disease, and (c) immune suppression giving rise to long term infections such as pneumonia.

In brief, the acceptance of cancer chemotherapy does affect nearly every part of the body and mind in numerous ways. There are better procedures as cancer treatment than chemotherapy with drugs. The holistic remedies are safe, nontoxic, natural, and effective. Alternative methods of healing to eliminate cancer have none of the adverse side effects invariably connected with allopathic medicine's synthetic chemotherapeutic agents. Anagen alopecia is the least of the side effects burdening the body by cancer chemotherapeutic agents. My advice is to avoid them at all costs.

Table 6-1 presents a list of cytotoxins that assuredly produce hair loss in the form of anagen alopecia that strikes sometimes within a week of taking the first chemotherapeutic agent. The efficacy of antineoplastic agents to kill cancer cells is well established. But in their effectiveness, they frequently kill other cells and tissues, including the whole person.

The listed drugs in **Table 6-1** bring on baldness for both men and women. They disrupt either cell cycling, cell growth, or the production of a specific component of hair.

TABLE 6-1

Cancer Chemotherapeutic Agents Proven to Cause Anagen Alopecia

Footnoted numbers refer to the clinical journal research papers referenced at the chapter's end which discuss characteristic effects of the listed cytotoxic agents utilized for cancer therapeutics

As indicated in the journal articles, anagen alopecia is among the many adverse side effects

Amsacrine[6]
Bleomycin[7]
Chlorambucil (rare)[8]
Colcemid[9]
Cyclophosphamide (Cytoxan®)[10]
Cytarabine (Ara-C®)[11]
Dacarbazine (DTIC®)[12]
Dactinomycin (Actinomycin D®)[13]
Daunorubicin (Daunomycin®; Cerubidine®)[14]
Dichloromethotrexate[15]
Doxorubicin (Adriamycin®)[16]
Endoxan[17]
Etoposide[18,19]
Fluorouracil (5-FU®)[20]

Fludarabine[21]
Floxuridine (FUDR®)[22]
Hexamethylmelamine[23]
Hydroxyurea[24]
Idarubicin[25]
Ifosfamide[26]
Lomustine (CCNU®)[27]
Mechlorethamine (nitrogen mustard)[28]
Melphalen (Alkeran®)[29]
Methotrexate[30]
Mitomycin (Mutamycin®)[31]
Mitoxantrone[32]
Nitrosureas[33]
Procarbazine[34]
Triethylenethiophosphoramide (Thiotepa®)[35]
Vinblastine (Velban®)[36]
Vincristine (Oncovin®)[37]

Why Cancer Chemotherapy Produces Baldness

The efficacy of anticancer agents and other cytotoxic chemicals is based on their ability to target and kill cells undergoing excessive and malignant subdivision *(mitosis)*. Since normal body cells have a slow turnover but most cancer cells are rapidly dividing, the cell poisoning drugs are relatively specific for cancer cells. Yet, certain normal body tissues which have naturally rapid turnover too, such as bone marrow, gastrointestinal mucous membranes, and hair matrix, must also be affected. As with abnormally growing and mitotic cancer cells, these normal but rapidly reproducing organ tissue and scalp cells respond adversely to the major toxicities of any of the chemotherapeutic drugs.[38]

In the case of surrounding cells within a hair follicle, this manifestation of adverse reaction is in the form of anagen alopecia, the diffuse shedding of an actively growing hair strand in its anagen phase that is the cause of baldness from drug cytotoxicity. The poisoned hair follicle lets go of the implanted hair strand and this individual hair falls out. The same thing tends to affect any of the anagen hairs. With catagen hairs floating in a state of resting dormancy and telogen hairs on their way out anyway, it's probable that the patient receiving chemotherapy will be losing most of his or her head hair and maybe similarly anagenic-phased hairs of the beard, axillae, pubic area, chest, legs, arms, eyebrows, and lashes. Head hairs, being most frequently in a phase of mitosis (replication), are more sensitive to the cellular poisons for cancer.

Thus, many chemotherapeutic agents are designed to attack cells in their most active phase of replication, namely DNA synthesis and mitosis.[39,40] Unfortunately, these poisons affect the growth and metabolism not only of malignant cells, but also of normal cells involved in the process of active replication.[41] Among all affected cells the hair follicles are most sensitive and mitosis in the hair matrix is suppressed so that hair synthesis gets impeded, which gives rise to hair fibers with fewer cells per unit length. Such hair is thin and fragile, and breaks off almost as soon as it issues from the follicle.[42]

The degree of hair loss depends on a number of factors. They include (1) the chemotherapeutic poison employed, (2) concurrent application of other agents that can cause alopecia, (3) drug dosage, (4) frequency of use, and (5) the route of drug administration. High-dose intravenous (IV) therapy results in complete anagen alopecia in a short time, whereas drugs given orally cause less alopecia, irrespective of the total dose used. Some oncologists have written that anagen alopecia starts approximately two to four weeks after the initial course of chemotherapy.[43] Others have stated that baldness arising from cytotoxic agents characteristically begins one to two weeks after the initial toxic chemotherapeutic dose and is most apparent at one to two months after the initiation of chemical treatment.

For complete clarification as regarding baldness that takes place from ingesting cytotoxic drugs, please recognize that its official medical name worldwide is *alopecia medicamentosa* and the description of such hair loss is *anagen effluvium.* It results from direct toxic insult to the rapidly dividing cells of the hair matrix. Some root sheaths die and others form weak, constricted hair shafts which then break upon growing outward and reaching the follicular opening to the skin surface.[44]

Because anticancer drug-induced hair loss is generally transient and not life-threatening, most oncologists have not been greatly concerned about their patients' baldness phenomena. On the other hand, the suffering patients tend to fear hair loss as among the most dreaded side effects of cancer chemotherapy even with knowing that it's potentially reversible. Because of such fear, immune systems of such patients have been adversely affected. Not only do the cytotoxic agents produce immune suppression for the patients, baldness does as well.[45]

Inadequate Measures Against Chemotherapy-Induced Alopecia

Some oncologists have been recommending the application of ice packs placed on the scalp prior to chemical therapy. The concept of such a practice is that ice placements will be useful by slowing scalp blood flow thereby reducing the effects of chemicals on the skin of the head and theoretically lessening the amount of lost hair. But such scalp hypothermia by cold applications has not shown great efficacy.

The hypothermic procedure could be applicable for some drugs with a short initial distribution phase and a rapid fall in blood plasma concentration during the first thirty minutes after infusion of the cytotoxic agent. Yet, this procedure is not recommended for use in tumors with high prevalence of scalp metastasis as in leukemia and lymphoma, because it may prevent delivery of the chemotherapeutic agents. In addition, disease could recur after scalp hypothermia for a patient who had an underlying mycosis fungoides (an eczema-like skin cancer) without other evidence of disease.[46] Such an increase of scalp metastases has been seen in some patients with breast carcinoma who had applied cold applications to the scalp.

The use of a scalp tourniquet in the prevention of chemotherapy-induced alopecia has been tried. In this technique, a tightly inflated pneumatic tourniquet with increased pressure above the systolic arterial pressure, is placed around the scalp at the hairline for ten minutes before, during, and twenty minutes after the cytoxic drug infusion.[47,48] Results with scalp tourniquets are poor. They cause headache and nerve compression.[49]

Doses of 1600 IU per day of alpha-tocopherol (vitamin E) administered for seventy-two hours before infusion have been tried to prevent alopecia medicamentosa, but the results remain unconfirmed by two prospective nonrandomized trials.[50,51]

Observed Hair Strand Pathology Produced by Chemotherapy

After patients have received cancer chemotherapy and do contribute their fallen hairs for microscopic examination, certain observed pathologies are observed in the hair. The *in vivo* exposure to individual chemotherapeutic agents produce various hair strand alterations.[52] With methotrexate taken as a prototype,[53] the microbiologist sees a decrease in the diameter of the hair bulb and its attached skin (keratogenous) zone. This reduction change takes place four to six days after a single dose of methotrexate or other cytotoxic agents. As the hair recovers with the elapse of time, growth of the matrix resumes and the shaft produced within the next two to five days shows up with a small constricted section. As the hair grows, the constriction moves to the hair's end (distally); with repeated doses of chemotherapeutic poison, however, successive constrictions of the hair shaft appear at the beginning (proximal) part of the hair strand.

These hair shaft constrictions from cancer cytotoxin ingestion are called *Pohl-Pinkus marks* and are similar to Beau's lines of the nails.[54] (*Beau's lines* are transverse grooves in the nail plate caused by various systemic and local traumatic factors plus nutritional deficiencies. For example, lack of the mineral nutrient zinc shows up as grey lines on the fingernails and toenails.)

Total scalp loss from cancer chemotherapy occurs with high doses or even low doses (5 milligrams times three) of methotrexate accompanied with the more dangerous impairment of kidney function.[55] Methotrexate has also been known to produce a unique change in blond hair called the *flag sign*. Here, multiple doses of methotrexate produce dark bands alternating with the patient's normal blond color in scalp hair, eyebrows, and nasal hairs (cilia). Its mechanism of pathology involves direct effects on the outer skin (epidermal) melanocytes stimulating melanin production.[56,57]

When nitrogen mustard gas is used as a chemotherapeutic agent, the oncologist performs a gaseous intra-arterial perfusion, and this causes an unusual localized baldness in the areas of distribution of the injected vessel.[58] Swelling of the skin and redness develop along with ulceration on the scalp. Following this, by the twelfth day after cytoxic ingestion, the hair falls out in the involved area. Histological evaluation of the cancer patient's scalp at that time of hair fallout shows follicular swelling and an absence of oil (sebaceous) glands and hair shafts. They disappear from the scalp but often return later after the chemotherapy is completed.[59]

People who suffer from cancer and require chemotherapy will probably be exposed to cytotoxic agents that are quite severe. The real life-threatening ones consist of vinblastine (Velban®), doxorubicin (Adriamycin®), actinomycin D, methotrexate, vincristine, cyclophosphamide (Cytoxan®), mercaptopurine (Purinethol®), nitrogen mustard (Alkeran® and Mustargen®), Diethylstilbestrol or DES, and others. All of them induce serious side effects. All of them are destructive not only to cancer cells but also to vigorously subdividing normal cells such as hair follicles.

If chemotherapy is to be continued as an integral part of cancer treatment, a means of preventing hair loss or to quickly restore hair growth to the bald head had to be found. Finding a baldness prevention program even with the use of cytotoxics was the object of numerous investigations over a long time. German university medical professors and oncologists participated in the research, and they did find an antidote to hair loss from chemotherapy. Proven are the topically-applied shampoo, gel, hair mask, and liquid preparations brand-named, *Thymu-Skin®,* which protect hair against the assaults of cytostatic cancer agents and other toxic drugs.

The following chapter will give some insight into the placebo-controlled, double-blind studies that followed development of the topical prevention modality for baldness even with a person's ingestion of cytotoxic chemicals.

CHAPTER SEVEN

How to Stop Baldness from Cytotoxic Chemicals

Sometimes it seems as if eagles are the only ones proud to be called bald. Dowling Stough, M.D., clinical assistant professor of dermatology at the University of Arkansas, suggests that there is a psychological root for being uncomfortable with baldness. Especially for the cancer patient who must take cytotoxic chemicals, hair loss upsets that person's need to fit in.[1]

"Having hair isn't necessarily an issue of vanity; it's an issue of being comfortable in society," Dr. Stough says. "When we lose our hair, it's no different than losing teeth or even a limb. We fight it and make adjustments, but we want to regain what we've lost: our previous appearance."

"We live in a time when appearance is important, and hair is a prominent accessory," says another dermatologist, Diana Bihova, M.D., clinical assistant professor of dermatology at New York University School of Medicine. "Baldness can cause an insecure self-image professionally and socially."[2]

How Many Cancer Patients Go Bald?

The current slogan among cancer therapists is: "Get cancer and go bald!" It's the most common observable characteristic of those unfortunate people who are directed to take chemotherapy for cancer.

Certainly anyone who loses his or her hair to cytotoxic chemicals applied as cancer treatment must be devastated by the experience—for two logical reasons: (a) the psychosocial stigma of appearing so very different from everyone else, and (b) the life-threatening aspects of needing cytotoxic drugs for a deadly disease. When suddenly one grows bald from taking chemotherapy, there's no denying that cancer has invaded the body. One need only to look in the mirror to be reminded.

In 1998, as has been the case for each of the prior years of the 1990s, about 1,040,000 new cancers will be diagnosed. Over 80 percent of these affected people will die from their disease. Cancer is the second leading cause of death in the United States, and accounts for 10 percent of the total annual health care cost.[3] In the year 2000, malignancies are anticipated to overtake heart disease as the most frequent killer of Americans. The educated estimate of both the National Cancer Institute and the American Cancer Society is that among the U.S. populace one out of three people will develop some form of cancer in their lifetime.[4]

Chemotherapy Is Used Even with Its Toxicity

Four basic cancer treatments are offered by the orthodox medical establishment: (1) surgery to remove the tumor, (2) radiation to shrink or kill remaining cancer cells at the tumor site, (3) chemotherapy to poison cancer cells in the bloodstream, and (4) narcotic drugs or steroids for pain in the disease's later stages. Collectively and by themselves, these four conventional treatments have an outrageously high failure rate that's greater than 80 percent and rising.[5]

Although chemotherapy has the worst ratio of success as a source of remission (never cure) for cancer—between 4 to 6 percent, it's still the most popular form of conventionally administered cancer treatment.

Chemo means "chemical" and *therapy* means "treatment"; thus *chemotherapy* is the administration of powerful, toxic drugs made from usually synthesized chemicals which are intended to kill cancer cells. They are most often given by intravenous infusion, but are sometimes taken orally. The recognized methods by which chemotherapy is standardly administered are:[6]

- *Orally,* by mouth as tableted pills, capsules or in liquid form (known in abbreviated medical jargon as *per os* or just "PO");
- *Intravenously,* by either being injected into a vein as a syringe and needle shot (IV push) or as a slower fluid drip ("IV" or "IV drip");
- *Intramuscularly,* by being injected into a muscle in the arm, buttocks, or thigh ("IM");
- *Subcutaneously,* by being injected beneath the skin ("SQ");
- *Intra-arterially,* by being injected into an artery ("IA");
- *Intrathecally,* by being injected directly into the spinal fluid ("IT");
- *Intracavitarily,* by being injected into the pleural space (lung) or into the abdomen (for fluid accumulation).

Typically chemotherapies are given by oncologists over a stipulated-period of time rather than in a single large dose. Since the drugs are intended to kill fast-growing, unwanted cells such as cancer cells, they also kill the body's fast-growing desirable cells such as hair follicles. As explained in the previous chapter, that's why hair strands fall out from chemotherapeutic use. The scalp's many growing and subdividing follicles in anagen phase are damaged or killed by the cytotoxins. Worse, chemotherapeutic drugs also severely depress the immune system at a time when a strong immunity is most crucially needed.

While the chemotherapy may possibly inactivate cancer cells up to 6 percent of the time, invariably it makes life for the patient a veritable hell on earth usually ending in death sooner rather than later.

In some small way certain members of the medical profession have finally come to recognize this illogical usage of cytotoxic agents by the cancer industry. (More workers in the industry make a living from cancer than the number of patients who find it necessary to take treatment for it.) Editorializing in the *New England Journal of Medicine,* two physicians—nononcologists—who teach at the Harvard School of Public Health have called for a shift in research, from just strictly cancer treatment to the more appropriate aspect of prevention.[6]

The Incidence of Cancer Death

Since President Nixon's announced "War on Cancer" in 1970, there's been no progress toward preventing the dread disease. Consider the following figures: From every demarcated group of 100,000 people who came down with cancer in 1990, 202 of them died from the disease. That's one in 500. Assuming the average individual has an eighty-year life expectancy, the chances of dying from cancer during those eighty years becomes 80 in 500, or about one in six.[7] When Richard Nixon declared his "cancer war", the odds of death from any kind of malignancy were one in *twelve.*

To avoid the terrible side effect of baldness, cancer patients sometimes just refuse to take the cellular toxins which comprise each one of the various chemotherapeutic agents. They don't accept their oncologists' advice and, attempt to ignore the disease. Spontaneous remissions can sometimes occur, but rarely.

There are five dozen or more readily available and highly successful natural and nontoxic anticancer therapeutic alternatives to cytotoxic drugs such as nutritional supplementation, Haelan 951, shark cartilage, Carnivora®, Essiac, 714X, antineoplastons, hydrazine sulfate, iscador, macrobiotics, Gerson therapy, and DMSO therapy. Unfortunately, the majority of cancer patients have not learned about these choices.

The nonusers of conventional cancer therapies may undergo no hair loss but possibly they'll die of cancer. The users of nontoxic and natural alternative methods of healing cancer undergo no hair loss and possibly they'll live long and well even in the face of cancer. Each patient must choose his own way to approach treatment of the disease.

Cancer chemotherapy never leaves the patient's hair unscathed. For example, as described in Chapter Six, methotrexate produces a unique change in blond hair known by oncologists and dermatologists as the "flag sign": dark bands produced in the damaged hair strand alternate with the normal blond color. There is also a direct effect on the skin's melanocytes which stimulate hair pigment production. Any new hair that grows in after the chemotherapy ends often is of a different color, shape, or texture, and these changes may persist for the recovering cancer patient for several years.[8]

How German Cancer Clinics Preserve Patients' Hair

Seeing the distress that his clinic's cancer patients were undergoing from receiving chemotherapy—more from baldness than from the awful nausea and vomiting they experienced—the compassionate medical systems analyst, Professor Doctor Claus O. Koehler, Ph.D., former department head of Medical and Biological Informatics at the German Cancer Research Centre in Heidelberg, Germany, had his associates investigate the topically applied thymus gland extract to stop hair loss. I visited with Prof. Dr. Koehler at his Heidelberg research center department during my October 1994 trip to Munich to meet with cancer surgeon Ulrich Fink, M.D. With Dr. Koehler I discussed results that his staff had experienced in using the superb hair-preserving product which had been researched by Guenther H. Klett-Loch, President of the Mannheim-based company, Thymu-

Skin Cosmetic. After undergoing numerous formulation improvements during the course of its development, this relatively new product derived from an extract of the calf thymus gland, was given the internationally registered trade-name *Thymu-Skin®*.

Prof. Dr. Koehler reiterated, ''Loss of hair, especially for female patients, is an additional stress factor which does not support and definitely hinders the success of their cancer treatment. Immunological defenses of the body are diminished by the added stress of hair loss.''

The oncological colleagues of this research center department chief conducted hair-preservation studies on one hundred forty-four patients treated with the somewhat mild cytotoxic agent 5-fluorouracil and on one hundred seven patients who were administered the more potent Adriamycin. None of the cancer patients received both of these drugs. The malignancies treated were cancer of the stomach, lungs, kidney, pancreas, breast, prostate, esophagus, colon, and the lymphoma known as Hodgkin's disease.

The World Health Organization (WHO) scores hair loss according to five levels or degrees:

in *level zero* (0), no change in the hair's appearance occurs;

in *level one* (1), a slight thinning with minimal (reversible) hair loss is seen;

in *level two* (2), a noticeable thinning shows up with moderate (reversible) hair fall;

in *level three* (3), a patchy baldness with areas of bare scalp becomes apparent, but it is reversible;

in *level four* (4), total irreversible hair loss has taken place.

Using these measurements, statistician Prof. Dr. Koehler concluded that subjects applying *Thymu-Skin®* to their heads a week or more before they were treated and all during therapy with the mildly toxic 5-FU chemotherapeutic agent experienced good success in the prevention of hair loss. Their head hair was preserved without any sign of falling among 88 percent of the patients. The people receiving the more cytotoxic ADR agent exhibited less but still impressive benefits—a saving of head hair occurring for 72 percent of these Adriamycin-treated patients.

A Multi-Centered Study of Chemotherapeutic Hair Loss Prevention

Similarly, Professor Doctor of Medicine and Doctor of Pharmacology Niels Peter Luepke, M.D., Chairman of the Division of Pharmacology and Toxicology at the University of Osnabruck, Germany, carried out an off-premises multi-centered, carefully monitored clinical trial of *Thymu-Skin®* to see if it was effective in preventing hair loss when cyto-static agents were employed. None of the doctors or patients knew who was receiving thymus extract or a dummy product which looked, smelled, and felt the same. Prof. Dr. med. et Dr. pharm Luepke combined cancer patients from three German university hospitals: Munich, Hanover, and Mün-ster. His total placebo-controlled, double-blinded study pop-ulation involved three hundred seventeen patients who received a variety of cytotoxic agents for different cancers. These cytotoxic drugs consisted of 5-fluorouracil, etoposid, cis-platin, Adriamycin, and two others.

In analyzing his data, Prof. Dr. med. et Dr. pharm. Luepke saw some gratifying results. Of the Munich University Hos-pital study, in which sixty-three patients with malignancies involving carcinoma of the breast, colon, rectum, and sig-moid, 76.2 percent were prevented from going bald despite their having received aggressive cytostatic chemotherapy.

In the Hanover University Hospital study, cytotoxic drugs were administered to ninety-six patients suffering from a broad spectrum of malignant diseases. Success using *Thymu-Skin®* was achieved by 41.1 percent who showed no hair loss whatsoever; 17.8 percent had a quick and total reversal of their alopecia effluvium; 26.8 percent had only minimal hair loss; 14.3 percent underwent moderate hair loss.

In the Münster University Hospital study, 158 patients

had received powerful cytostatic-combined chemotherapy for overcoming predominantly stomach cancer or esophageal carcinoma. All the treated patients had turned bald! When given quantities of *Thymu-Skin®,* 108 or 68.4 percent exhibited quick and total reversal of the alopecia. The balance of fifty patients showed continued minimal or moderate hair loss.

I emphasize again that all of these studies conducted by Prof. Dr. med. et Dr. pharm. Luepke, as stated by him, definitely were placebo-controlled and double-blinded. Neither the patients or the doctors knew in advance which products used were the placebo and which were the hair restorative. Since they conform exactly to the recognized scientific method, such double-blind, placebo-controlled investigations are important in the annals of hair preservation or restoration. When Dr. Luepke broke the investigation's product code and discovered who used the active formulation of *Thymu-Skin®,* he and his colleagues learned why fully 80 percent of their patients experienced no alopecia of any kind. Only 20 percent had some hair loss; whereas the alopecia totalis rate in patients given the inactive formulation showed hair loss that was three times higher.

In summary, a clinical research report written by oncologist and pharmacologist Neal Peter Luepke, M.D., Ph.D., published in the January 1990 issue of the *German Journal of Oncology,* discussed a randomly organized, multi-center, double-blinded, placebo-controlled study conducted in university clinics in Munich, Hanover, and Münster. Dr. Luepke's investigation was for purposes of testing if the local application of a complex thymus extract accompanying cancer treatment could influence the loss of hair as a secondary effect of cytostatic chemotherapy. Prof. Dr. med. et Dr. pharm. Luepke wrote:

> In the study, 317 patients particulary with cancer of the breast and the gastrointestinal tract, which were treated with various cytostatic drugs were examined. Positive effects on the development of alopecia during cytostatic chemotherapy were observed during the use of *Thymu-*

Skin® preparations. The patient's beneficial responses depended upon the aggressiveness of their therapy. The most positive effects were achieved during cytostatic therapy for mammary carcinoma or malignancies in the large intestine and the rectal area.

According to these observations, the use of *Thymu-Skin®* preparations during low- to medium-range cytostatic chemotherapy schemes were useful in decreasing alopecia.[9]

A 94 Percent Prevention of Chemotherapy-Induced Hair Loss

In the Department of Surgery at the Ludwig Boltzmann Institute for Clinical Oncology in the Vienna City Hospital of Vienna, Austria, oncological surgeon Prof. Dr. med. Helmuth Denck, M.D., and his associates Prof. Dr. med G. Alth, M.D., Dr. med. G.M. Wallner, M.D., and Dr. G. Baumgartner, Ph.D., performed a study using *Thymu-Skin®* initially on twenty-seven cancer patients, then seven months later increasing it to forty cancer patients, mostly women. They had been administered a variety of mild or moderate cytotoxic agents which included the following:

- the standard CMF-regimen combining cyclophosphamid (Cytoxan® or Endoxan®) + methotrexate + 5-fluorouracil (5-FU);
- Novantrone (MXO) alone or combined therapy with platinol (DDP) or oncovin;
- another combination of cyclophosphamid (5-fluorouracil + DDP + Endoxan);
- Carboplatin monotherapy
- 5-fluorouracil monotherapy

The success rate for those Viennese cancer patients who received *Thymu-Skin®* as the prevention mechanism for chemotherapy-induced hair loss was 94 percent. The patients receiving *Thymu-Skin*® demonstrated the World Health Organization hair loss level of 0. In contrast, only 78 percent of the cancer patient control group receiving a placebo saved their hair. They demonstrated a hair loss level of 2. In his final report, Prof. Dr. med. Helmuth Denke wrote:

> By consequent of the local application of *Thymu-Skin*® products, there is a 16 percent lower frequency of hair loss when compared to the control cancer patients. The local application of *Thymu-Skin*® over a complete observation period of nineteen months showed no undesired side effects.

Chemotherapy Doesn't Have To Mean Baldness

The unrooting of one's hair does not have to be the inevitable accompaniment to cancer cytotoxic agents or other poisonous drug usage. While an ingested drug-induced baldness certainly is the common and distressing side effect of some widely used therapeutic chemicals, the situation has finally been changed for the better.

Hair contributes greatly to physical attractiveness and to body image, and so alopecia may result in decreased social interactions that are devastating to an affected individual's psyche. As the threat of anagen alopecia can cause some patients to refuse potentially remedial or medically proven adjunctive chemotherapy, the prevention, reduction, or elimination of this disconcerting side effect of baldness can enhance patient compliance to chemotherapy.[10,11,12]

CHAPTER EIGHT

Present Alopecia Treatments for Men and Women

The Incidence and Ages of Hereditary Baldness

Alopecia hereditaria or *androgenetic alopecia,* (hereditary hair loss), commonly known as male pattern baldness or MPB, may be found in sufficient degree to be of cosmetic significance in about 12 percent of all European, North American, South American, and Australian men as young as age twenty-five. In the other age groups, 37 percent of these bare-scalp males are in the vicinity of thirty-five years old; 45 percent are around forty-five; and approximately 65 percent have turned age sixty-five. Baldness increases somewhat thereafter for more elderly males, with age being a major factor in MPB. Consequently, male pattern baldness in the minds of the public at large is definitely associated with steady progress toward old age.[1]

Androgens, the usual scientific term collectively employed by medical personnel to describe the male sex hormones, cause MPB in genetically predisposed individuals. As discussed briefly in Chapter Two, the genes for this bare scalp trait are inherited equally from both the father and mother's sides of the family. The extent of baldness and age of onset vary from family to family and from one person to another within the family.

Since a man may inherit genes for MPB from either or both of his parents' ancestors, he may be more bald at a given age than either his father or his maternal or paternal grandfather or uncles. Or, he may inherit baldness genes from only one side of the family—the other side lacking this hereditary trait. Thus, this nongenetically affected man may be less bald than any of his male forebears at a comparable age.

Even the baldest scalp due to MPB contains tiny follicles that produce almost visible (not quite invisible) hairs. The hope of users of the broad-ranging and diversely advertised methods of hair growth is that the particular method being espoused will make it possible to keep the follicular roots in the anagen phase of growth. Continued encouragement sees those follicles sprouting abundantly thick new hairs. Yet, we must accept a bareheaded truth: it's extremely unlikely that a significant amount of hair will ever be grown on a bald scalp when that baldness has been caused by *alopecia hereditaria*.

Women, too, sometimes confront a problem with pattern baldness. The condition, female pattern baldness or FPB, is associated with thinning of the hair as one grows older. This may become pronounced at middle age or later. It's not related to any disease but seems to be the same type of condition as found in men. FPB may resemble that of MPB, but the front hairline remains for a woman and some thinning at the top of the scalp often becomes apparent to observers (see **Drawing 5-2**).

The Incredible Shrinking Follicle

Almost none of the topical and internal therapies offered by conventional allopathic medical doctors and none of the remedies importuned by hairdressers and/or cosmeticians work to permanently restore hair growth or prevent hair fallout. The lists of esoteric cosmetic remedies for hair loss are too extensive for commentary about each. The subsections which follow offer information about several of the legitimate medical/surgical treatments by dermatologists, reconstructive and plastic surgeons, and other health care professionals. Minoxidil as a potential source of temporary hair growth will be briefly discussed.

The bald truth about hair restoration is that most men and many women are subjected to the incredible shrinking follicle—from receptors on the hair follicle itself which have become activated and suddenly sensitive to the alchemy of the hormone dihydrotestosterone (DHT). Over time, the action of DHT causes each of the many hair follicles to atrophy (shrink). This is opposite to what happens inside a man's prostate gland. There, DHT causes hypertrophy (expansion) of those cells comprising the prostate gland. While the prostate's cells expand and join to produce benign prostatic hyperplasia (BPH), the hair follicle cells follow their own state of shrinkage and shutdown. Thus, the hair strands the follicles have given rise to get let go and fall out.[2]

Cosmetic procedures and products advertised as producing more head hair are supposed to stop this action of DHT, but seldom, if ever, does that happen. That's because every single hair on the head has a genetic blueprint detailing what will happen to it. The gene that determines whether someone will be susceptible to androgenetic alopecia is found in the autosomes, the nonsex chromosomes that occupy every cell of the body. The follicle does remain alive if connected to a good blood supply which may successfully nurture it, but over time the capillaries shrink from their nourishment, and the follicle grows smaller and eventually dies.[3]

Surgical Procedures to Produce More Head Hair

Specialists in skin and scalp preservation using techniques of dermatology sometimes can perform wonders to replace the dying and dead hair follicles with live transplanted ones.

This section will discuss certain surgical procedures performed on the scalp to produce more head hair.

Medical books declare outright that no therapy of excellence is known for male pattern baldness or female pattern baldness, although transplants from hairy to bald areas have been effective when performed either by reconstructive and plastic surgeons or skilled dermatologists who specialize in the different procedures. Hair transplantation is a surgical operation which in the past has carried the risk of infection, often has been painful, and frequently remains unsightly until the scabbing wounds disappear.

Hair transplants aren't any quick, or cheap, fix. In one of the techniques, punch grafting, plugs of hair-bearing skin are taken from the back of the head and placed on the top. Women with diffuse, thinning hair usually are not good candidates for this procedure. Between thirty and one hundred plugs, each containing about twenty hairs, are transplanted in a session. "The scalp can only take a certain number of insults," says John F. Romano, M.D., clinical assistant professor of medicine at New York Hospital-Cornell Medical Center in New York City. "Usually, several sessions are needed for punch grafting. Each session is separated by a few months of healing, which may involve some itching and swelling and temporary crust formation at donor and receiving sites. There could also be an artificial or mismatched doll's hair look at first," advises Dr. Romano. This result can actually become embarrassing to the patient with transplanted hair.

The cost for transplanating hair plugs is anywhere from $20 to $50 per plug and is almost never covered by American health insurance. Hair transplants are considered to be unreimbursable cosmetic surgery. Still, hair restoration surgery has grown from a $190 million industry in 1991 to a $950 million industry in 1997. It's anticipated to top $1.1 billion in 1998, largely because of major surgical advancements made during the past five years. Most of these advancements were introduced by members of the International Society of

Hair Restoration Surgery (ISHRS), the largest professional organization in the field.

Advances in Hair Restoration Surgery

Hair cloning, laser technology, and mega-graft sessions are among the projected advances in hair restoration surgery. Since alopecia affects two in five men and one in four women in the United States, hair restoration surgery is a growth industry for this country's dermatologists. It's become one of the most popular elective operations for American men.

Dom Unger, M.D., a plastic and reconstructive surgeon, originated the concept of hair transplantation in the early 1800s. Small pieces of hair follicles taken from the scalp (hair grafts) to correct hair loss have been carried out with varying success since 1893. In the early 1900s, hair grafts of the eyebrows, hand, scalp and other areas were being performed in different parts of the world, not only for hair growth but also to rid an area of unwanted hair. The Japanese began single hair grafts for eyebrow reconstruction in the 1930s, followed by small, full-thickness hair grafts to correct alopecia of the scalp, eyebrows and mustache areas.

Norman Orentreich, M.D., a New York dermatologist, is credited as the "father of modern hair transplantation." In 1959, Dr. Orentreich developed donor dominance, a biological concept which states hair that grows in certain areas of the scalp is genetically encoded not to shed. It maintains that same characteristic when transplanted to a recipient site. This also means that a hair follicle transplanted from a portion of the scalp with thick hair will maintain its growth and will not take on the characteristics of the site where it is placed.

"Hair restoration surgery is more popular today because the product is better," said Robert Leonard, M.D., past president of the ISHRS. "Specialists no longer use the painful, bloody techniques of the early 1980s where large plugs of hair follicles were moved from one area of the scalp to another, often resulting in a 'corn-row' or 'toothbrush' effect. Today, we are able to transplant single hair follicles for a softer, more natural-looking hairline.''

New techniques of plugging in hair are based upon the concept of hair economics, which posits that a limited supply of hair exists with demand increasing as the supply decreases over time. Specialists need to develop a strategy or ''blueprint'' of hair restoration based on prediction of future hair loss for an individual. ''The hair restoration specialist and patient work as partners to achieve desired results,'' said Dr. Leonard, during our interview. ''In this way, hairline transplants performed at an early age are not 'isolated' by future hair loss creating uneven and false-looking hairlines later in life.''

''Our specialty's specific function makes the most out of the hair that is left by either moving remaining hair or reducing bald scalp,'' said James Vogel, M.D., immediate past president of the ISHRS. ''The art of the specialty is knowing how to create a natural hairline by placing hair follicles in the appropriate areas with the appropriate densities.''

Taking advantage of new microsurgical techniques, the health care professionals specializing in hair transplants use fine needles to move grafts of one to three hairs. Compared to plugs, smaller grafts mean less scarring and a more natural, feathered look. The operation takes three to five sessions. Transplanted hair usually falls out, then regrows within six months.

In another surgical technique known as scalp reduction, the surgeon removes some of the bald skin and stitches together the remaining hair-bearing skin. As much as half the bald area can be reduced using this procedure, which is often employed at the same time as hair transplantation.

Tissue expansion is also employed by the hair specialists. Using saline-filled bags placed under the patient's hair-bearing areas and flap surgery in which wide strips of hair-bearing scalp replace removed bald scalp, they perform these other surgical procedures as well.

Although hair restoration surgery is still challenged by images of the past, dermatologists who have become today's hair specialists predict it will continue to grow in popularity as advancements progress in the field, and temporary topical remedies such as minoxidil fail to provide expected results.

According to a recent study, furnished to me by Drs. Leonard and Vogel, minoxidil provides a full head of hair in only 5 to 10 percent of cases, and moderate hair growth in only 15 to 20 percent of cases. In clinical trials of women ages eighteen to forty-five with mild to moderate degrees of hair loss, just 19 percent reported some moderate hair regrowth, while 40 percent had minimal regrowth after using the product for eight months.

Minoxidil Attempts to Produce Hair

Minoxidil, manufactured and distributed by The Upjohn Company as its brand-named hair-producing product Rogaine®, is an antihypertensive pharmaceutical. Originally developed for reducing high blood pressure, nowadays minoxidil is more often applied topically in solution strengths averaging 2 percent to grow hair on bald heads. But minoxidil has been considered of questionable value among dermatologists, since its daily users are trapped into applying the product twice daily forever. Even with faithful usage, significant hair regrowth doesn't happen.

Minoxidil results begin to show after five to ten months of use, first with the appeance of fuzz (vellus hairs), which is not regular hair. Gradually, real hair is supposed to take over. Once a person starts with the topically-applied drug, he or she must stay with it the rest of his or her life or the hair falls out. Side effects include scalp irritation and headaches in some people. ''I see using minoxidil as a kind of hold-what-you've-got program, rather than for growing a thick new head of hair,'' says dermatologist Dowling Slough, M.D.[4]

No one knows why minoxidil produces temporary hair growth. It's known to be a powerful vasodilator, but other drugs that dilate blood vessels do not promote hair growth. The jury on Rogaine® is hung—no decision as to its viability for hair restoration. The majority of men who have used it did not grow back hair. But some have arrested the process of losing their hair. For as long as one uses the drug at a cost of about $750 a year, it seems, the hair that's left on the head does remain there.

Taking oral minoxidil may result in more rapid hair growth, but cosmetically acceptable regrowth is seen in only 18 percent of patients. Adverse side effects connected with orally administered minoxidil include fluid retention, headache, depression, lethargy, palpitations and tachycardia. These toxic side effects make oral minoxidil an unacceptable mode of therapy for alopecia. Some dermatologists claim they achieve good results by combining topical minoxidil and topical retin-A, the antiaging skin formula.[5,6,7]

More Methods to Battle Hair Loss

In alopecia areata, dilute triamcinolone acetonide suspension (a steroid hormone) can be injected into the skin if the bald patches are small, but the hair-growing results are not lasting. Also, when receiving the drug, patients may need a low-sodium diet and potassium supplements to counteract its toxicity.

Another unusual treatment for alopecia areata is the experimental induction of a mild allergic contact dermatitis. Here, a topical irritant such as diphenylcyclopropenone (DCP) is applied to cause a scalp reaction in the form of itching, heat, redness, papules, macules, or blisters, etc. While sometimes there's benefit, if you try it, you won't like it!

Because the size of the market for hair-loss treatments is mind-boggling, additional possibilities to disguise bare scalps are numerous. Here are a few more possibilites:

- Other than simply ignoring the problem, wigs and hairpieces are used. They are among the safest routes. Good ones are expensive but, if properly matched to one's hair, they are virtually undetectable.

The International Society of Hair Restoration Surgery condemns wigs or hair additions and topical camouflaging agents—as the medical doctors refer to hairpieces—because they require continuous investment for cleaning and/or replacement as natural hair grows and its color changes. The executive committee of the ISHRS says, ''The overall cost for a person to purchase and maintain hair additions beginning at age thirty-five and ending at age seventy is an estimated $70,000, while topical remedies require an estimated long-term investment of $12,600. In comparison, the estimated cost for permanent hair restoration surgery ranges from $8,000 to $30,000 depending upon the number of surgical procedures required over the course of, a one-and-a-half to two-year time period.

''By the time sufferers see a hair restoration specialist, they have already learned that to have a full head of hair from Rogaine® or hair additions requires a lifetime of expense and hard work,'' say the ISHRS officials.

- Cosmetics that color the scalp and make the thinning of hair less obvious are another way to go. They are safe, but must be applied regularly.
- Hair weaves involve weaving artificial hairs with real ones, but they do present an alternative option. Sometimes this process backfires and the real hairs can get tugged out by the hair weave.
- Devices that fasten to the scalp can be risky because synthetic hair implants may cause infection and scarring.
- Glues and suction cups used to hold hairpieces in place can lead to irritation.
- Wig snaps woven into existing hair may pull out the real hairs as sometimes happens with hair weaves.
- Wires and small steel spikes that are buried in the scalp to be used as hairpiece anchors may bring on infection and scarring.

Hair-Growth Requiring No More Drugs, Rugs, or Plugs

For men and women, who've been beset by baldness relating to alopecia totalis, alopecia universalis, alopecia adrogenetica, and some additional forms of alopecia, or for those folk who face baldness from their need to receive cancer chemotherapy or other drug treatment causing alopecia medicamentosa, the advent of new hair growth and prevention of hair loss finally is at hand. No more drugs, rugs, or plugs are needed.

Thymus gland extract that comes from calves already scheduled to be butchered into veal chops overcomes baldness when formulated with certain herbs and nutrients and applied to the scalp. If manufactured into the four *Thymu-Skin®* follicular restoration products, Hair Treatment, Hair Mask, Hair Gel, and Hair Shampoo, all old or new baldies become blessed with a single hair regrowth program that's comfortable and works. This combination of ingredients is not a drug but rather a cosmetic sold over the counter and without any prescription required.

Thymu-Skin® is an externally used series of hair products made from specially purified, biologically active calf thymus extract combined with various botanicals such as aloe vera, nettle and birch, along with vitamins A, B, and F (unsaturated fatty acids), plus other healthy immune-assisting ingredients. In Germany, the combination of substances is formulated into a pleasant smelling shampoo and a cosmetically acceptable hair lotion, gel and hair mask. Only two of the four products are needed together: the shampoo and one of the other three. Its formulation for human application as a cosmetic is approved by the United States Food and Drug Administration, the Canadian Health Protection Branch, and the German Federal Public Health Office *(Bundesgesundheitsamt),* among other nations' regulatory agencies.

Of the various *Thymu-Skin®* ingredients, Dr. med. Thomas Rabe, professor in the Department of Gynecology and Endocrinology at the University of Heidelberg, Germany, advises, "The product's main therapeutic factors are the enzymatic hydrolized GKL thymus peptides, the biological activity of which has been proven in multiple clinical trials. In addition there are further important phytochemical proteins including birch or nettle extracts and aloe vera, among others."

Prof. Dr. Rabe has conducted extensive studies with *Thymu-Skin®* for the reversal of female patterned baldness in women. His patients had brought their health difficulties for treatment at the University of Heidelberg gynecology and endocrinology clinics.

One such woman, Lotte Krammer, age forty-two, an aerobics instructor from Ludwigshafen, Germany, suddenly was struck by acute hair fallout directly after she underwent a permanent wave and hair set at a beauty salon. Within four weeks of having her hair waved permanently, all of Lotte's hair was gone. It just fell out.

She consulted with many medical specialists for treatment. The last one she looked to for help was Dr. Rabe. Results of the patient's physical examination were normal, but her family history included an older sister and brother who had lost hair as they advanced in age. A scalp biopsy specimen taken of Lotte by Dr. Rabe showed "miniaturization of hair follicles and a mild perifollicular infiltrate." Microscopic examination of scales from her scalp revealed no fungus infection, indicating that her scaling was probably caused by seborrhea (excess sebum).

Most significant is that women who exercise frequently and vigorously like this aerobics instructor, undergo virilization, a process in which secondary male sexual traits are acquired from adrenal gland dysfunction. Lotte Krammer had developed acne and some of her breast tissue had been lost over time. Her acute hair loss might be another manifestation of virilization, especially after the trauma of permanent waving which could produce scalp scarring. Also, this woman's family history of baldness points to a genetic predisposition. Hairs her doctor examined microscopically were thinner than normal and sharply tapered at the end, suggestive of androgenetic alopecia.

However Dr. Rabe's evaluation was that his patient's problem came from the waving lotion and shampoo used in her former hair salon. In beauty salons, shampoos are usually purchased in concentrated form, and water without antibacterial agents is added at the salon. It's been reported in the medical literature that *Pseudomonas* infections can be induced from the use of such wash water. This happened to two people who went to the same salon within one week. The preservatives in individually purchased bottles of shampoo are usually sufficient to protect a person from infection. But that may not be the case when the shampoo is in concentrated form.[8]

This was suspected as the hair loss circumstance for Lotte Krammer—that a microorganism may have produced the problem initially. When Dr. Rabe saw her alopecia no infection was present, but Lotte's lack of hair was already well established. His treatment was not dedicated toward eliminating any kind of pathological microbe but rather to reactivating his patient's dormant hair follicles. They had stopped functioning. (See **Photographs 8-1, 8-2, and 8-3** for a description of Dr. Rabe's treatment.)

When advising beauty salons on how to prevent infections among their clients, there are four recommendations put forth by the Center for Disease Control and Prevention (CDC):

(1) All solutions should be mixed fresh each day, with unused solutions discarded at the end of the day;
(2) Containers for diluted products should be wide-mouthed and easy to clean;
(3) The containers should be washed, rinsed, and dried at least once during the day:
(4) The containers should be rinsed with 70 percent alcohol and allowed to dry at the end of each day.

Permanent Wave Solution

The other hair salon complication for Lotte Krammer may have been the permanent wave relaxer used on her hair.

The two major types of relaxers are the sodium hydroxide type and the guanidine hydroxide type. The pH of the sodium hydroxide or lye type of straighteners can vary between 13 and 14, which are exceedingly alkaline. These relaxers contain up to 3 percent sodium hydroxide and must be applied very carefully; otherwise, the cream can cause severe burning which must be neutralized with vinegar immediately. If the chemical is left on the hair too long, the hair shaft breaks, and the follicles may be damaged beyond their ability to regrow hair strands.

Newer lye-free straightening products contain guanidine hydroxide and lithium hydroxide. They are powerful chemicals still able to burn the scalp, eyes, and ears and must continue to be applied with care. Mild caustic burns of the scalp and neck secondary to relaxers are relatively common, especially with the alkali relaxers. The burns usually are not severe enough to require medical attention. More severe burns may result in blistering, but scarring rarely occurs and only palliative treatment is required. Still, permanent hair loss can occur because the burns, superficial or not, will possibly destroy the follicular unit and hair will be lost forever.

The cold wave process for permanent waving was invented in the 1930s. A solution of ammonium thioglycolate is applied to the hair, the disulfide bonds are broken, and the substance is neutralized with hydrogen peroxide, sodium perborate, or sodium or potassium bromate. The mechanics of a permanent wave take place during these four steps:[9]

(1) The hair is shampooed to permit water to enter the hydrogen bonds within the hair shaft to allow flexibility;
(2) the hair is then wrapped over rods or curlers;
(3) the hair is saturated with ammonium thioglycolate;
(4) after five to twenty minutes, the hair becomes limp, is neutralized, and hardens into the new shape around the rollers.

Every time a permanent wave is performed, some of the disulfide bonds do not reform. For this reason, hair that has had a permanent wave applied or has been processed is less strong, resilient, or elastic than when it is untreated. The cuticular scales fail to return tightly in place, thus leaving the hair a little more porous with each procedure.

How Lotte Krammer Quickly Restored Her Hair Growth

Lotte Krammer stopped her baldness by restoring new hair strands within nine months of starting daily applications of all four *Thymu-Skin®* products (Hair Gel, Shampoo, Hair Mask, and Revitalizer lotion). (see **Photographs 8-1, 8-2, and 8-3**). It was the extracted calf thymus gland material in each of the four products that reversed her hair loss problem.

The ingredients in *Thumu-Skin®*, most especially its externally applied thymus gland extract, herbs, and vitamins, are nutritional substances readily taken internally as dietary supplements. Many such dietary supplements exist for improving hair appearance, stimulating hair growth, and preventing hair loss. These nutritional ingredients for oral ingestion are the subject of the next chapter.

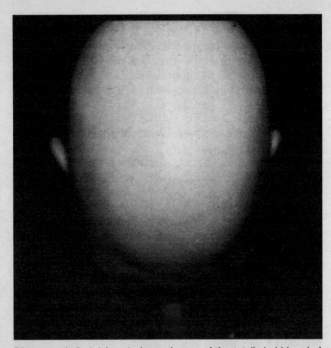

Photograph 8–1 (above) shows the top of the totally bald head of Lotte Krammer, age forty-two, an aerobics instructor from Ludwig-shafen, Germany. Permanent waving at a beauty salon performed two years before was the trigger for her hair loss which occurred within four weeks of the perm. The woman had been trying to regrow hair by consulting doctors and cosmeticians but to no avail. She is seen here in mid-1993.

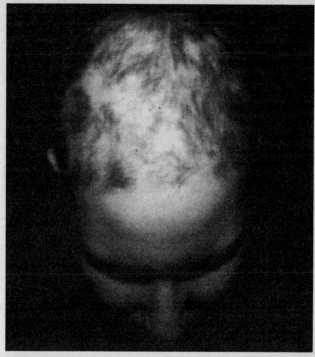

Photograph 8–2 (above) shows the top of Lotte Krammer's head with some restored hair growth just three months following the start of her daily applications of *Thymu-Skin*®.

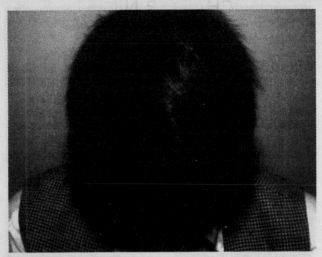

Photograph 8–3 (above) shows the top of Lotte Krammer's head sporting a full crop of bushy hair nine months from the day she began faithful applications of the various formulations of *Thymu-Skin®*. The main hair-growing ingredient in the product is refined extract of the calf thymus gland.

CHAPTER NINE

Using Dietary Supplements to Prevent Hair Loss

Answering readers' questions which appear in the "Man to Man" column for the May/June 1997 issue of *Natural Health* magazine, senior editor Bill Thomson responds factually to the following query:

"I m thirty-nine, and I m going bald around my temples and on the top of my head. I'd like to think I don't care, but it's bothering me a lot. Is there anything I can do?"

Editor Thomson replies: "If you eat a high-fat diet, cut back on the fat. Many generations of Japanese men had thick hair, but in the last half-century as they began to adopt a fattier diet, some have started losing it. It turns out that soyfoods (a staple of the traditional Japanese diet) block the formation of DHT (dihydrotestosterone), a male hormone associated with hair loss. Try eating more soy and seafood and less fat."[1]

That's good advice! In the next chapter I will discuss a nutritious fermented soybean drink imported from China, but this chapter discusses enhanced nourishment for hair follicles and the body overall from ingesting dietary supplements. Hair health can be improved by consuming quantities of vitamins, minerals, thymus glandular extract, ginseng's ginsenocides, and other edible items. Taking optimal nutrition is an important means of physiologically encouraging greater hair growth on the head to achieve the termination of balding. Hair follicles react postively or negatively to what a person eats. Readers of this book have adopted a motto. In our minds, we shout with an emphatic voice: *Bald no more!*

Going Bald from Poor Nutrition

The non-nutritious fare served by fast-food restaurants is a major source of hair loss for both adult sexes. The edible garbage taken into one's body from consuming chemical additives, free radical pathology, excessive fats, overly fried and overly sugared "fast food" offered by commercial establishments does more than bring on cancer, heart disease, and other forms of slow death. Far worse is that the fast-food restaurant's junk food products cause baldness from prolonged malnourishment of the head's hair follicles.

Crash dieting and following of fad diets too stringently are culprits contributing to baldness, as well. This kind of bad eating produces frail hair that breaks off and falls out more easily (at least temporarily). Crash diets possess too few daily calories. Fad diets often exclude essential nutrients. If a person lacks protein, carbohydrates, the normal amount of fats, or certain vitamins and minerals, his or her hair's health will surely be affected.

Because the hair is comprised mostly of protein (known as *keratin),* it needs an input of appropriate amino acids and other proteins to stay healthy. Insufficient amounts of this vital protein nutrient can lead to a temporary loss of color and texture. The resulting thin, dry, lusterless hair sheds easily. A protein deficiency will produce the faster onset of hair telogen (the termination phase of a hair strand's growth cycle when it falls out.) If not corrected, permanent rather than temporary baldness develops from the onset of a constant telogenic phase in the hair cycle.

Carbohydrates and fats contribute to the normal activities of growing hair, so they shouldn't be eliminated from the diet. Carbohydrates provide energy that helps the body use protein and improve cell growth in the hair follicles. Fats are important to the sebaceous (oil) glands, which produce the sebum that naturally conditions hair. Sebum, itself is an oil fat, specially composed by the body to keep the hair follicles lubricated.[2]

Vitamins for Nourishing the Scalp and Restoring Hair

Although deficiencies in the vitamin B complex and vitamin C can cause problems for your hair and scalp, **vitamin A** is exceedingly important for having healthy hair. Too little vitamin A in the diet will lead to one's hair becoming dry and dull. Eventually the individual hair follicle's root lets go so that the hair bulb dies off or forms a cyst around itself. This arises from the dietary deficiency of vitamin A that usually is self-created.

Vitamin A deficiency tends to stimulate the outer layer of the scalp's skin layer to grow over the mouth of each hair follicle near the accompanying sebaceous gland. This overgrowth then obstructs the follicle's opening, slows hair development, and keeps sebum from flowing properly.

Because the keratin cells continue growing, they may form "plugs" as well that block the hair from coming out and cause the sebaceous glands to wither. Hair loss must be the eventual result of such blockage.[3]

Certain members of the **Complex B Vitamins** hold vital positions in the hierarchy of hair restoring nutrients. Four particular B vitamins which are absolutely necessary consist of PABA, biotin, pyridoxine, and inositol. Each has a connection to hair growth.

PABA (para-aminobenzoic acid) has been known to reverse premature graying when taken as an adjunct to the diet. The dosage of PABA recommended by the author of *Prescription for Nutritional Healing,* James F. Balch, M.D., to take for restoring hair or for returning graying hair to its former color is 50 mg twice daily.[4]

Biotin is not manufactured by the body because it gets plenty of it from diet or from friendly bacteria (probiotics) living in the intestines. If only egg whites are eaten or intravenous feedings are received for extended periods, a biotin deficiency that causes hair loss might be experienced. Still, research shows that hair regrows when biotin is taken in a program of nutrition against alopecia areata, or patchy baldness. Biotin is known to bind testosterone in the hair follicle instead of allowing the testosterone to bind with the protein receptors that turn it into DHT. Because less DHT is available to "attack" the follicle, hair loss slows down or stops. Nutritional supplements, creams, shampoos, conditioners, and hair sprays containing biotin are readily available for use, often from the health food store (as are all the hair-growing items in this chapter).

Pyridoxine (vitamin B-6) participates in sixty enzymatic reactions that metabolize amino acids and essential fatty acids. Its deficiency results in adverse changes of the nervous system, mucous membranes, skin, hair, and nails. The dosage of this vitamin to stimulate hair growth or improve its luster is 50 mg three times daily.[5]

Inosital helps to stimulate follicular growth of hair strands following acute alopecia as a result of toxic metal syndrome, drug reactions, severe allergic response, child birth complications, and other body dysfunctions. Nutritionist Shari Lieberman, M.A., R.D., coauthor of *The Real Vitamin and Mineral Book*, suggests that the proper dosage of inosital for hair restoration may be 100 mg two times a day.[6]

Ascorbic Acid (vitamin C) invariably gets included in hair restoration formulas. Even conventional dietitians who are unversed in nutrient supplementation, frequently agree that vitamin C plays a role in health of the skin, hair and nails. When combined with the **Bioflavonoids** in a dosage of 500 to 5,000 mg in divided doses, vitamin C promotes hair growth by improving blood flow to the scalp.[7]

Other Nutrients Beneficial in Restoring Hair

Zinc taken in a dosage of 15 to 50 mg is credited with halting hair loss and stimulating new growth in some cases. At any rate, besides the mineral zinc, at least **one multi-mineral supplemental tablet or capsule** taken daily is good nourishment for the scalp.

Tissue Salts such as the homeopathic remedies **Calc. Phos., Kali. Sulph., Nat. Mur.,** and/or **Silicea** are recognized as helpmates in correcting hair-loss problems. The suggested homeopathy dosage is three 6X tablets dissolved under the tongue (sublingual) twice daily.

Additional nutrients which have been advantageous in the past for treatment of falling hair include **Folic Acid, Pantothenic Acid, Copper, Iodine, Magnesium,** and **Sulfur.** Adjunctive to these recognized scalp feeders, an individual's supplementation could include **Unsaturated Fatty Acids** such as **Evening Primrose Oil, Flaxseed Oil,** or **Salmon Oil; Niacinamide,** a derivative of **Niacin** (vitamin B-3); **Alpha Tocopherol** (vitamin E); **Coenzyme Q**[8] (ubiquinone); **Dimethylglycine** (DMG); **Kelp;** plus the necessary amino acids **L-Cysteine, L-Cystine,** and **L-Methionine.**[9]

Herbs have value for stimulating hair growth. The leaves of the herbal, **Nettles,** have been used for centuries. The Nettles are rich in vitamins A and C, and a wide range of minerals including **Iodine, Silicon,** and **Sulfur,** all valuable for improving hair growth. The internationally known Swiss herbalist, A. Vogel, M.D., suggests that a formula for hair loss should include one part nettles leaves, one part onion and one part 70 percent alcohol. The nettles and onion should be soaked in the alcohol for several days, then the resulting solution massaged into one's scalp followed by shampooing the hair. Carry out this procedure daily, he recommends.

There are two more herbs helpful for hair growth. **Rosemary** is employed for cleansing the scalp and exciting hair roots, and **Sage** is designated as a safeguard against falling hair.[10]

Raw Thymus Glandular Substance Taken Internally

Any informed hair growth specialists who utilize nutrition as part of their hair treatment programs usually place thymus gland extract at the top of their protocols for patients who suffer from baldness. Dr. James Balch recommends that a person trying to restore hair growth should ingest raw thymus glandular substance (500 mg a day) because it stimulates immune ability at the same time it improves the functioning of hair follicles and endocrine balance. He comes from the school that believes baldness is an autoimmune disease, and one primary way to offset the problem is by boosting one's immune system.

As previously mentioned, I have researched the subject of thymus gland extract as the antidote to hair loss among eight prestigious medical centers, each of them an integral part of a German university teaching hospital in such cities as Frankfurt, Munich, Heidelberg, Münster, Hanover, Osnabrueck, Darmstadt, and Vienna, Austria. What I've learned is that any informed physician—at least those located in Europe—knows and recommends the diverse immunity-building benefits of taking raw thymus glandular tablets, capsules, sublingual drops or powders internally as nutritional supplements. These additions to one's food supply may be purchased in almost any health-food store or by mail order from nutrient supply houses.

Calf thymus extract is one example of a substance employed for a remarkable anti-aging treatment program. This entire method administered by ''youth doctors'' has been built up around cellular therapy. In cell therapy, the physicians and other therapists employ glandular extracts taken from young or fetal animal organs and administer them in injectible and sublingual form to attain the prolongation of youth and the extension of life for their patients. It's been reported by the press that cell therapy has been taken by such notable actors as Kirk Douglas, Robert Cummings, Marlene Dietrich, Ronald Reagan (before he became president), Lillian Gish, and numerous other prominent people, even including Pope Pius XII.

Stresses that Damage Hair Follicles

Part of the problem for hair follicles is that they respond adversely to situations of stress that occur when the mind or body comes under pressure, bears the burden of tension, gets overtaxed, or labors in a state of fatigue. Stress has a psychological, physical, chemical, and biological effect on a person's total physiology. Chronic stress, especially, produces a steady drain on the energy supply to all functioning cells, and the result must invariably be cellular malfunction.

Hair follicles are particularly prone to reacting poorly in the presence of subnormal bouts of energy production because they are vigorously subdividing repeatedly and continuously. More than any other type of somatic cells, except perhaps for bone marrow and gastric mucosal cells, hair follicles perpetually are renewing themselves—they push up individual hair strands toward the surface mouths of their skin orifices by means of this ongoing subdivision. An abundance of energy is needed to move along these newly formed hair strands. When follicles malfunction, they stop subdividing, go into a situation of withdrawal which becomes prolonged quiescence, and then begin to atrophy. Such damage eventually results in the circumstance recognized as hair loss, which actually has derived from the harmful effects of prolonged stress on the immune system.

I have mentioned that some of the more technically advanced health professionals—including Dr. James Balch—consider baldness to be an autoimmune disease. Dermatologists and other researchers have discovered that, for example, the body's production of its own cancer-fighting cells, including nature, killer cells, is inhibited by chronic stress. Distress stops normal function in cells, tissues, organs, and additional body parts. Another example of immunological weakness resulting from ongoing stress presents itself by the realization that people catch colds, experience migraines, or activate gastric ulcers when they are under a lot of pressure to perform.

Job stress is increasing to worldwide epidemic proportions. It's affecting massive numbers of people, mostly those with occupations involving tensions, pressure, and decision-making. This news, which makes sense, is reported by the International Labor Organization of the United Nations (ILOUN).

The ILOUN goes on to say that all over the world sleep disorders are one of the main consequences of stress on the job. President Bill Clinton is among those growing numbers of Americans who find it hard to get a good night's sleep. Hillary Rodham Clinton admits that the hectic schedule in the White House has put sleep on hold for her husband and herself. "It's the stress," she says. The president has complained of periods of sleeplessness that have his close aides worried.

Job pressures among ordinary Americans are estimated by the Labor Department to cost the U.S. economy $255 billion annually through reduced productivity, increased compensation claims, prolonged absenteeism, higher health insurance premiums, and greater amounts of direct medical expenses.

It's well understood that 80 percent of all illness and disease is stress-related. What's less known is that hair loss happens from stress, too. Many incidences of baldness could be eliminated by doing away with situations of stress at home and in the workplace. The three best-selling drugs in the United States, tranquilizers, painkillers, and gastrointestinal remedies, were developed to counter stress. Two-thirds of all visits to family physicians stem from stress. It's the root problem for anxiety, alcoholism, headaches, hypertension, irritability, hair fallout, and many other common ailments.[11]

Adaptogens Are Nature's Answer to Stress

Nature's antidote to stress is a combination of herbal ingredients called *adaptogens*. The recently deceased reknowned Russian research pharmacologist and physiologist, Israel I. Brekhman, M.D., is the discoverer of adaptogens. Defined by Dr. Brekhman, an adaptogen is a botanical—a plant type with certain characteristics:

(1) it is nontoxic and safe for ingestion by animals, including humans;

(2) it increases the body's nonspecifc resistance by being stress-adapting;

(3) it tends to bring back to normal (homeostasis) any dysfunctioning body systems such as hair follicles. When combined, each adaptogenic plant builds on the therapeutic attribute of the others present in the nutritional formula to offer a kind of synergistic effect.

Early on, officials in the former U.S.S.R. recognized the efficacy of Dr. Brekhman's phytochemical (plant product) physiological breakthroughs which occurred before 1966. It was in 1968 that they formalized the term he had coined, *adaptogen*. Investigation by the Russian scientist and his team uncovered that adaptogens accomplish the following benefits in human and animal physiology. They:[12]

- increase protein biosynthesis;
- raise antibody levels (the blood titre) at immunization;
- elevate the body's enzyme synthesis by means of general endocrine stimulation;
- enhance mental work capacity;
- uplift physical work capacity along with performance and endurance;
- quench free radicals so as to prevent oxidizing pathology;

- improve eyesight, color perception, hearing, and vestibular functions;
- offer advantageous effects in the cardiovascular and respiratory systems;
- promote longevity;
- heighten the body's nonspecific resistance to various physical stressors such as toxins, excess cooling, overheating, altered barometric pressure, ultraviolet, ionizing, and cosmic radiation, and too much motor activity;
- elevate the level of sexuality and sexual performance;
- encourage the retention of hair strands by their follicles.

Ginseng Is the "King of Adaptogens"

Exhibiting a wide sprectrum of therapeutic effects, **Ginseng** in its three botanic forms of *Panax quinquefolius* (American ginseng), *Eleutherococcus senticosus* (Siberian genseng), *Panax ginseng* (Korean genseng) support immunity when the human organism is stressed. It favorably influences the hearing, sharpens the eyesight, increases night vision, helps further dynamic adaptation of the eyes, significantly improves color vision in color-blind people, increases physical and mental work capacity, encourages the retention of scalp hair, and does other good things for the body and mind. Botanists who know the field, consider ginseng to be the "King of Adaptogens".[13]

Dr. Brekhman and his associates had studied the effectiveness of adaptogenic plants on the basis of daily and seasonal changes in individuals as well as under differing environmental circumstances. He originated the new Western science of ecological pharmacology when he investigated the complex formulas found in ancient Chinese pharmacopoeia. Ginseng therapy comes from Chinese medical science, used for purposes of retaining youth, stamina, and sexual prowess. The heads of hair on even quite elderly Chinese males stay well-textured, black-colored, full and bushy when they take ginseng as a daily nutritional supplement.[14]

Any plant identified as ginseng is known to come from a broad family of botanicals, all shown to be effective for helping build energy levels gradually and without a stimulant effect. Thousands of clinical and laboratory investigations have demonstrated ginseng's benefits (four are cited below). It rebalances the body in innumerable ways, especially as the means of combating the damaging effects of stress. The plant is used throughout the Far East as a general tonic to neutralize weakness and give extra energy.[15]

Eliminate Hair Follicle Stress with Oral Ginsenocides

The active ingredients in ginseng which promote hair growth and other health benefits are thirty different chemicals, the triterpenoid saponins, collectively known as *ginsenocides*. They give the herb its stimulative effects on human physiology. Only the most advanced ginseng products made from the plant's root, stem, flower, and leaves contain these thirty different ginsenocides. The type of ginseng, the total ginsenocide content, and the ratio of the ginsenocides from the plant's root, stem, flower, and leaves determine the extent and degree of benefits available from the use of the herb. Some ginseng products are less potent than others because they are processed only from the plant's root, and contain just seven of the ginsenocides in their makeup. These produce an inferior therapeutic result.[16]

The botanic form of ginseng which works most effectively to eliminate stress on hair follicles and for enhancement of the heart, blood vessels, immune system, and memory retention for the brain has recently been discovered to be *Panax quinquefolius* (American ginseng). This North American ginseng has not been used for as long as the other two types and has been grown in the United States only during the last century. (Siberian and Korean ginseng have been employed for approximately 4,000 years.) Since North American ginseng shows the best therapeutic effects, however, Asians come to this country and buy whatever supply they can negotiate from American growers of the plant.

The Asian processors take these raw plants home to China, refine them into commercial products such as chewing gum, tablets, capsules, beverages, medicinals, powders, spantials, bakery goods, and other ingestible items, and then export these products back to Americans and Canadians. The world's best ginsenocide products arrive at our ports as "full spectrum," 100 percent pure ginsenocides made from North American ginseng. They are extracts derived from all of the plant, its root, stem, flower, and leaves.

Pegasus "Gold Medal Formula" Ginseng is the "king" of ginsenocide products, and the only type most suited to improving follicular strength. For enhancement of hair growth from the body's internal area outward, North American ginsenocides are the preferred product. The Pegasus formula is distributed through a toll-free number by BioTek Nutritionals, Inc. of Metairie, Louisiana. (See Appendix One).

Medical Studies Showing the Efficacy of Ginseng

Long suspected as arising from an autoimmune disease, an experimental double-blind investigation of baldness was carried out by clinical researchers among three groups of twenty healthy human volunteers to test this theory.

Among the sixty patients, each group was given capsules containing either 100 mg of aqueous extract of ginseng (Group A), 100 mg of lactose (Group B), or 100 mg of standardized extract of ginseng (Group C). All subjects took one capsule every twelve hours for eight weeks. Blood samples were withdrawn from them before beginning the treatment, at the fourth week and at the eighth week.

The ginseng extract standardized for a 4 percent ginsenoside content (Group C) was more active and created a greater immune stimulating effect than the aqueous extract of ginseng (Group A) which indicated a moderate immunological boost. The lactose placebo (Group B) showed no immune system stimulation at all.[17]

In an animal experimental study, ginsenosides were administered to mice at a dose of 10 milligrams per kilogram of body weight (mg/kg) for three consecutive days before immunization increased the animals' spleen plaque-forming cells, their antigen-reactive T-cells, their number of T-helper cells, and the splenocyte natural killer cell activity. The ginsenosides induced the augmentation of interleukin one (IL-1) by macrophages. Ginsenosides also partly restored the impaired immune reactivity by cyclophosphamide (a toxic drug) treatment.[18]

In a second mouse study, an aqueous extract of ginseng was administered orally to the animals for six days at a daily dose of 10, 50, and 250 mg/kg. The treated mice responded with enhanced antibody formation to challenges with sheep red cells. The effects were dose-dependent. Immunity increased as high as 50 percent with the mere elevated dose of ginseng.

Natural killer cell activity was increased as high as 150 percent. Ginseng showed two main therapeutic effects in the mice, an inhibition of stimulated and spontaneous lymphocyte proliferation and an enhancement of interferon production.[19]

A fourth ginseng investigation, this one conducted again with human subjects, proved that ginseng improved their immune system function. In an experimental double-blind study, thirty-six healthy volunteers received 10 ml of standardized ethanolic preparation of ginseng or ethanol placebo three times daily. After four weeks, subjects in the study group receiving ginseng showed a drastic increase in the absolute number of immunocompetent cells, with pronounced effect on T-lymphocytes, predominantly helper/inducers. Also their cytotoxic and natural killer cells were increased. In addition, they experienced a general enhancement of T-lymphocyte activation. No side effects were observed during the six-month observation period.[20]

Unquestionably, the taking of ginseng as a nutritional supplement is a practice that enhances the immune system.

If baldness comes from a malfunction in the immune system as discussed in the next chapter, taking the Pegasus "Gold Medal Formula" of full spectrum, 100 percent pure ginseno-cides that come from North American Ginseng is the way to go.

CHAPTER TEN

The Ultimate Nutritional Drink to Stop Falling Hair

In November 1996, Frederick "Fred" R. Williamson, age forty-six, a high school teacher living in Cleveland, Ohio, learned that he had been struck by testicular cancer (known medically as *seminoma*). His family physician came upon the potentially malignant growth while palpating Williamson's scrotal sac during a routine physical examination that he underwent each year. He did not take this news well, especially when treatments offered by both the consulting urologist and oncologist were surgical removal of the affected testis (an orchidectomy) followed by a long bout of chemotherapy. The two physicians could not promise that this procedure would be a cure.

Until his cancer diagnosis was made through a needle biopsy, an MRI (magnetic resonance imaging), and other medical examinations, the worst health problem this patient could recall having was the onset of baldness. From about age forty, Fred Williamson had been seeing bits of his brown hair floating down the shower drain, sprinkling the bedsheet, or caught in his comb and brush. He was balding at the crown and forehead, and hair loss had been causing him some anxiety. But now that cancer had struck, baldness, in comparison, was no problem at all.

Testicular surgery and chemotherapy were not what he wanted, so Williamson refused this conventional treatment advice and sought out alternative methods of healing. He went looking for safe, natural, nontoxic therapies. To find them, he attended health conventions and read extensively. Fred subscribed to numerous alternative health magazines, newsletters, and some clinical journals on holistic medicine. Among the many articles he read was a sizeable group that discussed anticancer nutrition. The chief nutritional remedy exhibiting success for reducing or eliminating hormonal and urogenital cancers of his general type was the Chinese use of a liquid fermentation product made from soybean proteins. There were at least twelve research papers published by U.S. Research Reports, Inc. describing laboratory and clinical studies carried out in the People's Republic of China.

Williamson learned that this beverage is so packed with micronutrients it actually reverses cancer and other degenerative pathologies such as emphysema, high blood pressure, blood dyscrasias, diabetes, heart disease, osteoporosis, arthritis, skin eruptions, and much more. It does taste awful, the medical journalist wrote, because this drink comes from soybeans, which offers an unmistakably pungent odor and distinctively cloying flavor. But the product's users, even those with serious health problems, feel elevated energy, less stress, a greater sense of well-being, inner peace, overall calmness, increased strength, much happier, and physically healthier overall. Medical papers and magazine articles have been published that furnishes this information.[1,2,3,4,5,6,7]

Best of all, 82 percent of the time (reported among fifty patients across the United States) their various disease processes went away. Fred decided that along with other nutritional supplementations such as taking ginsenocides and popping down nutrients, he was going to drink this fermented soybean product.

Fred Williamson Starts Drinking Haelan 951™

He contacted Haelan Products, Inc., located in Woodinville, Washington, and purchased a twenty-bottle case of the Chinese import. It's brand-named **Haelan 951**™ (see Appendix One for the company's address and toll-free telephone number). When the case of Haelan 951™ arrived, Fred Williamson followed directions and immediately started to drink an eight-ounce bottle per day half in the morning and half in the late afternoon. He did this religiously, and experienced a good response within a week. Since the cancer patient felt so marvelous—full of energy and good cheer—by the sixteenth day he ordered another case. A couple of weeks later he took delivery of a third case of twenty bottles, and then two more cases.

Williamson's daily drinking of Haelan 951*™* continued over a three-month period at which time he went for some more diagnostic testing. His physician was worried about him because he had refused conventional oncological treatment procedures and was self-administering for testicular cancer strictly with nutritional therapy.

When the laboratory test results came in, his family doctor expressed amazement. It was a Friday, March 14, 1997, that Fred Williamson learned he had no more signs of cancer. His cancer markers were normal. The testicular tumor had shrunk and disappeared. Another biopsy proved that the cancer was gone.

Believing that Haelan 951™ had brought him a new lease on life, Williamson elected to continue drinking the fermented soybean beverage as a means of cancer prevention. He wanted no recurrence, and he knew that elevating his immune system as much as possible was mandatory.

The Autoimmune Attack Upon Hair Follicles

According to numbers of American and European clinical researchers, Alopecia areata has been associated with other diseases, most of which are related to pathologies of the immune system.[8,9,10,11,12,13] Added to this, unusual associations with baldness include testicular atrophy or dysfunction as well.[14] Therefore, if he had possessed a fuller amount of medical knowledge, Fred Williamson, by manifesting immune system suppression and associated testicular dysfunction, could have considered his hair loss, starting at age forty, to be an early sign of some serious underlying health problem. In Fred's case, his baldness was associated with testicular cancer.

My belief, based on reports from dermatologists and a document search of medical journals from around the world, is that baldness reflects an autoimmune attack upon hair follicles. While other factors such as heredity, pollution, excessive androgens, stress, poor nutrition, toxic metals, and other sources of pathology bring on hair loss, medical science should classify baldness among syndromes of the autoimmune diseases. All indications point to baldness being an autoimmune disease.

An **Autoimmune disease** is the abnormal situation in which one's immune system incorrectly identifies "self" as "nonself" and executes a misdirected immune attack. Such a pathological situation is illustrated by the symptoms associated with rheumatoid arthritis, Type I diabetes, psoriasis, multiple sclerosis, myasthenia gravis, systemic lupus erythematosus, and forty other autoimmune diseases recognized by health care professionals. In these disease states, a person's immune system destroys his or her body tissues. Not counting those affected by baldness, from 5 to 7 percent of the American population is subject to autoimmune diseases, and a similar percentage of the afflicted prevail in other Western industrialized nations. The chance of one's experiencing an autoimmune reaction increases with age.[15,16]

Baldness has an immunological connection that becomes apparent when histologists look at alopecia-affected anagen hairs under the microscope. What they see in anagen alopecia are white blood cell (lympocytic) infiltrates and granulation tissue arising in response to chronic infection (granulomatosis). There is inflammation around the anagen hairs as well as within the hair follicle in the acute progressive stage of alopecia areata.[17] Immune system inflammatory cells, primarily CD4+ lymphocytes and other blood components known as Langerhans' cells, are present around the hair bulb (peribulbar) and blood vessel (perivascular) areas. The autoimmune attackers are present as well in the external root sheath which is lined with numbers of follicle cells (follicular epithelia).[18]

Histologists report observing three different patterns of hair follicle cellular degeneration in states of acute alopecia from autoimmune disease. These pathologies include local tissue death (necrosis), cell fragmentation (apoptosis), and dark cell transformation.[19] There are blood elements of the immune system actively engaged in a kind of cellular destruction of the hair follicles. These blood elements include mononuclear cells which infiltrate around the particular follicule being attacked in this autoimmune reaction. Moreover, specific cytotoxic T-lymphocytes attack a normal anagen hair bulb as if it is a protein substance foreign to the body (an antigen). Indeed, in Alopecia areata, HLA (human leukocyte antigens), specifically the HLA-A, HLA-B, HLA-C, and HLA-DR antigens are all expressed on anagen hair bulbs.[20,21]

These microscopic observations are further discussed in Chapter Eleven by dermatologists Desmond J. Tobin, M.D., Norman Orentreich, M.D., David A. Fenton, M.D., and Jean-Claude Bystryn, M.D.. They indicate that the incidence of baldness, especially Alopecia areata, is definitely tied to being an autoimmune disease. My conclusion is that correcting a malfunctioning immune system could possibly stop the ongoing occurrence of hair loss.

Boosting the Immune System Stops
Hair Loss for Fred Williamson

This very positive circumstance of eliminating falling hair happened for Fred Williamson. Five weeks after he received his verdict of a life free of cancer, the man underwent what could be described as a "eureka!" experience. As if a lightbulb began flashing in his brain, Williamson suddenly realized that excessive numbers of hair strands were no longer shedding from his head. He didn't see them lining the bathroom sink, floating down the shower drain, coating his pillow, attaching to his collars, or being caught by his hairbrush and comb. It seems that boosting the immune system by drinking Haelan 951™ stopped his hair loss completely.

Looking histologically at the autoimmune attack on the anagen phase hair follicle when mounted on a microscopic slide, this termination of hair loss is quite explainable. The immune system will have calmed down as a result of its return to normality. Cell death occurs now only to the outer root sheath keratinocytes, as in normal catagen. The circumscribed cystic change that had taken place in the suprabulbar region above the dermal papillae has stopped. The lymphocytes and granulocytes have been withdrawn, and inflammation has been dissipated from within the hair follicles and around the late anagen hairs. Cell adhesion molecules, which mediate cell-cell and cell-matrix interaction, have been withdrawn. Endothelial cells lining postcapillary venules are no longer present.[22]

The T-cells are not migrating to the hair follicles anymore, nor are they penetrating the outer root sheath basement membranes to interact with certain soluble inflammatory mediators such as ICAM-1 (intracellular adhesion molecule-1), ELAM (E-selectin), tumor necrosis factor-alpha and gamma interferon, and VCAM-1 (vascular cell adhesion molecule-1).[23] In brief, the immune system's responses to what it had conceived as exciting antigens have been neutralized.

Why does this immune system restoration occur? Because

there is excellent nourishment furnished to every somatic cell by a person's ingestion of concentrate derived from a patented fermentation process that uses the advanced proprietary fermentation process of bacteria number 951 yellow as the inoculum. The fermenting bacteria work on proteins which have been handpicked in China from over 10,000 variable soybean species. They are the very best that farmers from all over China can provide, for these soybeans are designated for medicinal purposes.

The Nutritional Components in Haelan 951™

The Chinese soybean drink is rich in selenium, zinc, vitamins A, B-1, B-2, B-12, C, D, E, and K, plus the amino acids alanine, arginine, aspartic acid, cystine, glutamie acid, glycine, histidine, isoleucine, leucine, lysine, methionine, nucleic acid, ornithine, phenylalanine, proline, serine, threonine, tyrosine, tryptophan and valine. (See **Table 10-1** for a summary of amino acids and their amounts in Haelan 951™.)

Plant chemicals (phytochemicals) are nature's illness-preventing ingredients furnished to animals—including humans. There are more phytochemicals per gram of bulk weight in soybeans than in almost any other vegetable or fruit. Recognizing the therapeutic value of soybeans, in 1996 the National Cancer Institute (NCI) invested nearly $3 millon to study the prime healing ingredient in them. Added to this United States grant the National Institutes of Health (NIH) spent another $20,000,000 in a research program to determine the therapeutic benefits of phytochemicals in the three particular plant foods: garlic, licorice, and soybeans.

TABLE 10–1[24]

Quantities of Amino Acids Present in 100 Ml of Haelan 951™

Alanine	47.3 mg	Methionine	14.8 mg
Arginine	33.8 mg	Nucleic acid	3.0 mg
Aspartic acid	6.6 mg	Ornithine	1.8 mg
Cystine	14.9 mg	Phenylalanine	22.7 mg
Glutamic acid	77.6 mg	Proline	11.4 mg
Glycine	33.4 mg	Serine	22.7 mg
Histidine	7.9 mg	Threonine	34.7 mg
Isoleucine	18.9 mg	Tyrosine	22.2 mg
Leucine	42.9 mg	Tryptophan	1.9 mg

In these government studies it was found that certain soybean components, the nine phytochemicals consisting of genistein, daizin, glycitin, acetylated daizin, acetylated glycitin, acetylated genistein, malonylated diazin, malonylated glycitin, and malonylated genistein, taken together or separately, block angiogenesis. **Angiogenesis** is the formation of new blood vessels, a process essential for the development of a tumor. In cancer production, the nine phytochemicals in soybeans inhibit angiogenesis even more effectively than does shark cartilage; only soybeans are much less expensive from which to make an anticancer beverage such as Haelan 951™. The soya phytochemical group called isoflavones exhibits the most powerful anticancer effects.[25]

Isoflavones are plant estrogens (phytoestrogens), that are about 1/100,000th the strength of human estrogen. Such weak estrogen activity is responsible for the anticancer effects of isoflavones in hormone-related cancer such as breast cancer. Estrogen increases cancer risk by binding to breast cells. Because they are so similar in structure to human estrogen, isoflavones can also attach to the receptors, effectively blocking human estrogen. But because isoflavones are so weak, they don't have the deadly effect that human estrogens do. The most widely used drug in breast-cancer treatment, tamoxifen, works in just this way.

In clinical studies testing the effect of soyfoods on cancer, Kenneth Setchell, Ph.D., professor of pediatrics at Children's Hospital and Medical Center in Cincinnati, demonstrated that regular soyfoods contain enough isoflavones to have a marked hormonal influence. Dr. Setchell fed a group of women 60 grams (g) of textured vegetable protein (TVP) daily and observed what happened to their menstrual cycles. After four weeks, the time between their cycles increased two to five days. Longer menstrual cycles mean a lower lifelong exposure to estrogen, which in turn lowers cancer risk.

Dr. Setchell then tested whether an Asian-style fermented soyfood such as is present in Haelan 951™ might have the same effect. He again fed the volunteers 60 g of Chinese soy beverage. ''It had an even bigger effect. It shifted the menstrual period an extra day,'' said Dr. Setchell, who has now been working with the aid of a financial grant from the NIH to study the physiological effects of the different soy estrogen compounds.

Studies of the factors leading to the occurrence of disease among large groups (epidemiological studies) reinforce the Setchell findings and suggest soy may help reduce rates of other cancers in addition to those of the breast. We know that the prostate benefits from a man's ingesting soyfoods, which not only includes Haelan 951™ but also miso, cooked soybeans, soy flour, soymilk, soy nuts, soy protein isolate, tempeh, tofu, and TVP (textured vegetable protein). All of these nutritional products may be found in natural health food stores, co-ops, some supermarkets, and by mail order. My suggestion is to eat as much soy as possible. Bake with soy flour, drink soymilk, and eat other soyfoods like tofu and TVP. In addition, a regular diet can be supplemented with a daily intake of two ounces of Haelan 951™. Make a concerted effort to add soy to the diet for purposes of illness prevention, perfect health, and to eliminate baldness that comes from immune system suppression.

Soybean seeds have been consumed by humans for thousands of years because they are rich in protein (35 percent) and their oil is of good nutritional quality. Most East Asians consume soybean seeds regularly from childhood, via a variety of soybean products. The incidence of breast and colon cancer in Asian people is considerably lower than in those living in Western countries,[26] who seldom eat soybean products. Additionally, vegetarians, who are also at decreased risk of breast and colon cancer, frequently consume soybean-based meat substitutes.[27] These epidemiological associations suggest that the consumption of soybeans plays a role in reducing breast and colon cancer risk.

In a significant animal study, researchers pointed out that ''carcinogen-induced mammary tumorigenesis [breast cancer] was inhibited by feeding the laboratory animals isoflavonoid-rich soy products.''[28] The same thing happens in women and men. The incidence of breast cancer and prostate cancer is definitely lowered by the ingestion of soybean concentrate such as Haclan 951™.

So particular phytochemicals in soybeans tend to reverse the occurrence of cancer and stop hair from falling out. Yet, while this ultimate nutritional drink may not stimulate the growth of *new* hairs, there is another substance—an animal acquired glandular extract—that does that rather well. I will discuss calf thymus extract combined with nutritional ingredients in the following chapter.

CHAPTER ELEVEN

General Therapeutic Effects of Calf Thymus Extract

Swimming around in each human being is a sea of antigens. It is a swarm of dangerous environmental invaders consisting of viruses; bacteria; cancer cells; pollens; molds, yeasts, and other fungi; protozoa, worms, and other parasites; toxic metals; chemical pollutants; radiation; plus natural and synthetic poisons threatening from without and from within, to potentially produce disease and death. The way people are able to survive periodic unexpected assaults on our health and life from these antigens is by use of an innate and acquired immunity!

The official definition of an **antigen** is any substance the body regards as foreign or potentially dangerous against which it produces an antibody (a defense). Because of this possible physiological derangement (a pathology), the immune system goes on to create quantities of antibodies. Sometimes the "natural poison within" is viewed with alarm by the immune system. Even if the poison could be considered "self," the immune system forms antibodies against the body's own components. These self-attacking antibodies are identified in medical science as *autoantibodies*.[1]

In Chapter Ten, I discussed the potential for baldness being an autoimmune disease—a derangement of the immune system in which the "self" fights battles against "self" and a person's body produces its own antigens of "self" (called *autoantigens*). From the Ronald O. Perelman Department of Dermatology at New York University Medical Center in New York City and the St. John's Institute of Dermatology at St. Thomas's Hospital in London, four of the world's most prominent dermatologists affirm that baldness develops from an autoimmune attack on hair follicles.

The research that proves these physicians' conclusion was supported by grants from the National Alopecia Areata Foundation, the Heckscher Foundation for Children, and the United States Public Health Service. What's stated in the dermatologists' clinical journal report is that in balding people, the physiology goes awry and forms antibodies against normal human anagen scalp hair follicles so that Alopecia areata results.[2]

Immune System Participation in Hair Loss

Direct evidence of abnormal immune responses to the hair follicles in patients with Alopecia areata was demonstrated by four dermatology researchers: Desmond J. Tobin, M.D., Norman Orentreich, M.D., David A. Fenton, M.D., and Jean-Claude Bystryn, M.D. They made observations about abnormalities in the blood circulating antibodies to the hair follicle antigens of sixty-six subjects. The blood of thirty-nine balding patients was compared to twenty-seven nonbalding controls by the Western immunoblotting technique. At the conclusion of their investigations, the dermatologists wrote: "These findings indicate that individuals with Alopecia areata have abnormal antibodies directed to hair follicle antigens, and support the hypothesis that Alopecia areata is an autoimmune disease."

They studied five types of antibodies to 6 M urea-extractable proteins of normal anagen scalp hair follicles. All of the tested Alopecia areata patients (100 percent) possessed antibodies to individual hair follicle antigens. This antibody reading was seen in the bald patients up to seven times more frequently than in the control subjects. Incidentally, among those controls antibodies were present in 44 percent, which indicates that potentially they were going to go bald sooner or later.

Based largely on the prior published reports of their dermatological colleagues, the investigating doctors made some significant statements regarding the immune system's participation in causing anagen hair loss:

- Alopecia areata is a systemic disorder.[3]
- Hair loss is associated with the presence of a lymphocytic infiltrate around or in hair bulbs.[4]
- Increased numbers of Langerhans cells (blood elements offering antigens involved in immune responses) are present within affected hair follicles.[5]
- Balding causes deposits of immune reactants around hair follicles.[6]
- Abnormal immunogenic molecule (thymulin) levels are found in individuals with Alopecia arcata. There is an expression of two classes of antigens, MHC class I and MHC class II, in the hair bulbs.[7]
- Any effective therapies for Alopecia areata have, as a common denominator, an effect on immune cells in the skin.[8]

The hair follicle antibodies labeled by immunologists as numbers 44, 47, 50, 52, and 105 kD, found in balding people, frequently direct themselves to antigens that are specific for hair follicles. These are the sites where the antibodies do their damage as misdirected protection. They don't selectively damage any other skin components—just hair follicles.

Of interest to note is that alopecia areata preferentially affects pigmented hair and spares white hair. When balding stops and the regrowth of hair tends to occur, such new hair is often initially white.[9] In addition, the hair pigment cells *(melanocytes)* may be selectively damaged both in affected hair bulbs[10] and in other locations such as the eyes of patients with alopecia.[11]

Role of the Thymus Gland in Immune System Reactions

White blood cells *(leukocytes),* seven thousand per cubic millimeter $(7000/ml^3)$ in one drop of human blood seen microscopically, have 27.5 percent of them consisting of lymphocytes, the main fighting troops of the immune system. The lymphocytes' job is to circulate through the blood and tissues to locate, trap, and destroy the threatening antigen invaders. Two types of lymphocytic cells exist: the B-cells (the B-lymphocytes) migrate from the *bone marrow.* (The "B" part of B-cells indicates the source is bone marrow.) The T-cells (the T-lymphocytes) migrate from the *thymus gland.* (The "T" indicates their origin is the thymus.)

T-cells develop into various specialized kinds of cells responsible for cell-mediated immune reactions. *Cell-mediated* means that rather than responding directly to the presence of antigens by producing antibodies, T-cells influence neighboring white blood cells, so as to turn on or turn off (mediate) reactions within the immune system.

One type of T-lymphocyte known as the T_4-*helper cells,* specifically induce the B-cells to "turn on" and respond to the presence of an antigen. They also stimulate another kind of T-cell, the *Natural Killer cells* (NK cells), to kill invading foreign cells by means of direct contact or by producing a cell poison (cytotoxin). In contrast, the T_8-*suppressor cells* regulate the immune response by "turning off" blood cellular activity. Under normal conditions there is a proven ratio of 1.8 T_4-helper cells for each T_8-suppressor cell.

Thus, a primary organ of the human immune system is the thymus, a ductless gland located deep in the chest under the breastbone. The thymus reaches its maximum size, relative body weight, during early childhood, and then begins to shrink. Shaped like a pyramid with many lobules, the superficial area of the thymus gland can be touched by tapping the top of the breastbone at the base of the neck.

If secretion from one's thymus is inadequate, it can be enhanced by ingesting quantities of glandular extracts made from the thymuses of calves. Such a glandular extract is referred to in medicine as a *protomorphogen,* and its medical application for body organ benefit is known as *cellular organotrophy* or just "cell therapy."

Besides taking the thymus protomorphogen orally, it can be injected intravenously (into a vein), intramuscularly (into a muscle), and subcutaneously (under the skin), or by sublingual (under the tongue) absorption. Easier still is topical (through the skin) application. Any of these methods of thymus extract self-administration are advantageous to the immune system. The most convenient method of application, is to massage thymus extract into the scalp. Such an action will preserve hair against possible fallout, perhaps regrow hair that's been lost, and simultaneously boost the immune system for the building of necessary blood system T-lymphocytes.

Why Thymus Protomorphogen Is Beneficial

An investigation performed at the National Cancer Institute (NCI) of the United States in the 1960s illustrates the benefit of using calf thymus extract as a protomorphogen for boosting any animal immune system (including for human beings). Into newborn baby mice possessing no thymus glands were implanted calf thymus tissues which contain the small peptide hormone known as *thymosin.* The added thymosin stimulated the animals' spleen and lymph nodes into making their own lymphocytes. These white blood cells are the major defensive and surveillance system of an animal's body and become extremely important in defending against disease and degeneration.[12]

American immunologists Allen Goldstein, M.D., and Abraham White, M.D., have discovered that thymosin in thymus gland extract is extremely active in stimulating the human immune system. In clinical trials, patients found to benefit from receiving thymus extract were those with genetic immune deficiencies. Thymosin proved itself useful in the treatment of cancer, since it restores one's cell-mediated ability to prevent malignancy.[13]

In the same manner thymosin holds off the aging process itself. The body's immunity definitely decreases with age as do the quantities of thymosin circulating in the blood along with the capacity of the aging human thymus to produce new T-lymphocytes. But, when extra supplies of thymic protomorphogen are added to someone's blood circulation, an increased resistance to most kinds of infections, cancer, and all manner of age-related deteriorative changes take place. In that way well-being and good health for any person are sustained over a much longer period of years.[14]

In a series of experiments performed in 1976, thymus protomorphogen as raw glandular extract was discovered to yield 200 mg. of active thymosin per 1,000 gm. of crude calf thymus powder produced by the azeotropic process. Cooking the glands or heat-treating the thymus tissue leads to complete loss of thymosin activity and therefore this preparation of active thymosin is distinctively dependent upon the method of preparation of the glandular material. Such a thymus extract used for two studies, first raised immune chemical competence of laboratory animals receiving it and second, showed clinically that human cancer patients taking the preparation also experienced a boost in their immune system abilities.[15]

Thymus glandular tissue prepared by the appropriate refining process that leaves active thymosin in the tissue and then gets ingested by a person in any manner, including its topical application, is a treatment of choice for many immune-related difficulties. Thus, application of calf thymus extract to the scalp of a person's bald head can bring large immune-boosting benefits.

Thymus Extract Neutralizes Self Against Self

It's believed by some dermatologists, and theorized by immunologists and other doctors, that baldness is an autoimmune disease in which self attacks self. To summarize the hypothesis: the balding person's own white blood cells are recognizing certain hair follicles not as normal body components but rather as foreign proteins which need to be eliminated. Knowledgeable dermatologists and immunologists who have done research in this area of hair loss have shown that the body's immune system turns various sets of hair follicles into autoantigens (body-produced antagonistic proteins), to which it responds by producing autoantibodies. These autoantibodies attack the autoantigens to bring about dysfunction, deterioration, and death of hair follicles. In fact, any part of the immune system may go haywire in this way, but it's particulary apparent among bald persons because one can see their autoimmune response in the form of hair loss.

When ingested in any manner such as being absorbed internally through the scalp, the thymosin in calf thymus extract seems to act as a normalizing or reducing agent in the body's creation of hair follicle autoantigens. It tends to neutralize the response of autoantibodies and stop the attack of self against self. Hair follicles will then no longer be set upon by components of the immune system. White blood cells appear to discontinue considering one's own hair follicles as enemies of the body. Thus, someone who absorbs extract taken from the thymus gland of a calf, lamb, or other natural source that's close in molecular structure to the human thymus, causes an immunological normalization or leveling off (homeostasis) to take place. This is the same way that cell therapy works.

The research team of an independent laboratory, Orpegen Pharma of Heidelberg, Germany, under the direction of Prof. Dr. Christian Birr, Ph.D., did research in this area. Orpegen Pharma determined the specific biological activity of the thymic preparation which is the major therapeutic component of *Thymu-Skin®*. This preparation contains essentially short peptides with molecular weights ranging from 300 to 1,000 daltons (a measurement scale used in biophysics). In his February 28, 1994 laboratory study report, Prof. Dr. Birr wrote:

The test substance [*Thymu-Skin®*] showed significant immunomodulatory effects on human lymphocytes. Peripheral blood lymphocytes were stimulated. . . . This increase in lymphocyte proliferation was accompanied by a dose-dependent rise of Interleukin-2 receptor expression and antigen density on T-lymphocytes.

In other words, the Interleukin-2 receptor of T-lymphocytes which regulates their activity, including their rate of reproduction is modulated by the tiny peptides in *Thymu-Skin®*. Dr. Birr's laboratory analysis confirmed what many German clinicians already suspected—that the very small molecules present in this evaluated thymus extract enhances human immunological function.

Thymus Extract Rejuvenates Against Aging

Published in the *International Journal of Thymology,* which offers exposure to "investigations pertaining to clinical immunology and endocrinology," an article stated that thymic hormones, as immunotransmitters, modulate the hypothalamic-pituitary-adrenal and hypothalamic pituitary-gonadal axes. The central nervous system is affected, so that active substances of the thymus gland influence the processes of aging. Using thymic materials derived from fetal thymic calf extracts or from very young bovine animals have rejuvenating effects. The article's four authors, representing both the Department of Biology and Genetics and the Department of Physiology of the Silesian Academy of Medicine in Sosnowiec, Poland, plus the Institute for Immunology and Thymus Research in Bad Harzburg, Germany, state:

Biochemical, morphological and sumicroscopic changes occurring as a result of the administration of the thymic extracts showed clearly a regenerating effect on all the examined tissue and organs, such as blood, thymus, peripheral lymphopoietic organs, liver, kidneys and lungs. The thymic calf extracts effect is the stongest one. It brings, for a short time, the organs of mature animals to the state corresponding to that of fetal life. The mature thymic preparations bring the aging organs to the morphological and biochemical state corresponding to that of young, healthy animals.[16]

Immune Dysfunction Aided by Thymic Protein

It is estimated that sixty-five million Americans suffer from a dysfunctional immune system. Among the manifestations of this disorder are a variety of diseases, such as AIDS, arthritis, asthma, allergy, diabetes, chronic viral infections, chronic fatigue syndrome, cancer, the yeast syndrome, and much more. Baldness is now recognized as one of those immune system diseases too. A large portion of immune dysfunction and suppression may be due to thymus functional deficiency, because the thymus gland plays such a pivotal role in initiating and regulating immune response.

Knowledgeable alternative and complementary health professionals have treated deficiencies involving the thyroid gland and other glands with physiologic replacements. I have previously mentioned whole thymus gland ground down and dried, or strained into liquid and injected or administered in capsules or sublingual drops as part of cell therapy.

By the very method of processing for cell therapy, such products are a conglomeration of thymus tissue, cell debris, fragments of thymus proteins, and thymus by-products. These extracts have been available for decades and have shown variable levels of effectiveness for various immune deficiencies and some specific medical conditions. In fact, one such fragmented thymus protein, the drug Thymosin, has been approved as an adjuvant treatment for hepatitis B in China.

Prior to the introduction of *Thymu-Skin®* for topical application on the scalp, thymic extracts have contained only fragmented thymic peptides, tiny proteins which showed only limited effectiveness. To attain full efficacy, a protein must have a specific shape with precisely defined transmitter and receptor sites. Such a protein has been developed, and this is discussed at length in the next chapter. Thymus peptides may be administered topically—even through the scalp—as well as the other ways previously described. All of the delivery methods for thymus extract provide the human organism with a variety of health-preserving benefits.

Thymus Extract Protects Against Degenerative Diseases

In another significant article published six months later in the same thymology journal, it was made clear by the authors that "thymic factors are useful for prevention and therapy of clinical entities such as carcinomas, autoimmune diseases, and immunological deficiencies as well as for endocrinological disorders."

Thymus peptides of the type present in *Thymu-Skin®* were designated as one of the long-acting agents with efficacy beginning within one month which offset autoaggressive disorders as occurs when a person's self attacks self.

In this second clinical journal article, it was shown, as well, that thymus peptides support T-lymphocytes in recognizing the tumor-antigens in cancer. Thymus enzymes are involved in decreasing malignant metastases. Other degenerative disease entities which respond to thymus extract in combination with enzymatic therapy are rheumatoid arthritis and viral infections such as herpes zoster and herpes labialis.[17]

In conclusion, the immunological advantages of regularly utilizing calf thymus peptides—their autoimmune neutralization effect and their immune system boosting benefit—in addition to their stimulation of hair growth—make calf thymus extract an extremely worthwhile product to use against particular degenerative diseases.

Thymus peptides furnish a triple harvest of good health. Plus, for the balding person, alopecia reverses from the application of calf thymus extract externally so that hair loss stops and hair growth begins.

CHAPTER TWELVE

Studies on Thymus Extract to Reverse Alopecia

In the autumn of 1978 when he was twenty-two years old, a newly graduated mechanical engineer, Dieter Norbert Kloss, of Darmstadt, Germany, suddenly was struck by the loss of hair from his head and various body parts. He experienced extensive hair loss all over, including total scalp hair elimination, cessation of beard growth, the fallout of eyebrows, and later he became denuded of hair in every other area—the chest, arms, legs, pubic region, and both armpits. Yet, this baldness changed dramatically for the better—fourteen years later.

The diagnosis for this young German engineer was *alopecia areata totalis* (loss of all scalp hair) and *alopecia areata universalis* (loss of all body hair). No medical reason for the disease ever was determined.

For a decade afterward, Dieter, with the help of his loving parents, sought out a cure—or at the very least, some cause—for his condition. Over time he took treatment with a variety of dermatological therapies: (a) multiple corticosteroid injections into the scalp, (b) steroids by mouth with their many adverse side effects, (c) skin allergens to distract the immune system away from hair follicles, causing him an awful itching rash, (d) night applications of the tar-like ointment anthralin which discolored his skin, (e) smearing on light-sensitive psoralen cream that was subsequently baked with ultraviolet rays, (f) various and diverse diets, (g) electronic stimulation to the scalp, (h) laser beams combined with scalp sensitization, (i) psychological counseling to reduce the obvious stress he was under, and (j) minoxidil as Rogaine® produced by The UpJohn Company when it first was introduced. There were other miscellaneous and innumerable barbershop and beauty parlor remedies tried by him too.

Traveling from hair-growing salons to clinics, hospitals, and medical centers and then on to the offices of general physicians, internists, dermatologists, plastic surgeons, and other specialists were of no avail for this young professional. By 1990 he had despaired of restoring his hair growth. Although he had been troubled for many years, Dieter Kloss finally did accept his fate of standing out from the crowd.

Thirteen years following the onset of his total scalp and body baldness, Kloss entered a free, dermatologist-supervised, university-sponsored, placebo-controlled, double-blind clinical study of the German hair-growing formula, later identified as *Thymu-Skin®*. He was among the group of several hundred patients who experienced great success by their raising new crops of hair on heads and bodies where they wanted it to reappear. It took nine months of cosmetic liquid application, but the investigation worked well for Dieter N. Kloss (see **Photographs 12-1, 12-2, 12-3,** and **12-4**).

A calf thymic preparation (thymus extract) containing multiple tiny molecular proteins (as described in Chapters Eleven and Thirteen) usually referred to by biochemists as *short-chain peptides* was the primary healing agent for the young engineer's baldness problem.

The hair-raising tale unravelling here is about the topically applied preparation known as *Thymu-Skin®* that excites dormant but living follicles to regrow hair. Moreover, it seems to stop one's own autoimmune attack of the hair follicles. *Thymu-Skin®* is verified as tested and valid in eight university medical centers throughout Germany and Austria.

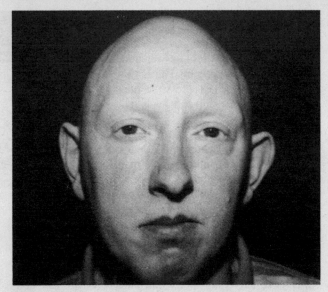

Photograph 12–1 (above) shows a Darmstadt municipal clinic patient in the autumn of 1993. After fourteen years of being totally bald (no head hair, beard, eyelashes or eyebrows, and denuded of hair on the rest of his body) this thirty-seven-year-old engineer, Dieter N. Kloss of Darmstadt, Germany, embarked on a daily program of applying *Thymu-Skin*® only to the bare scalp on the top of his head.

The Darmstadt Study of *Alopecia Areata Totalis et Universalis*

In Darmstadt, clinical studies were conducted during 1991 and 1992 which verified that this new hair preparation reverses certain forms of alopecia. In one of the smaller studies, Prof. Dr. med. Manfred Hagedorn. M.D., Medical Director of Darmstadt University Medical Clinic and Chief of the Darmstadt City Hospital Dermatology Department, and his able dermatology associate Klio Moessler, M.D., enrolled twenty patients suffering with *alopecia areata*

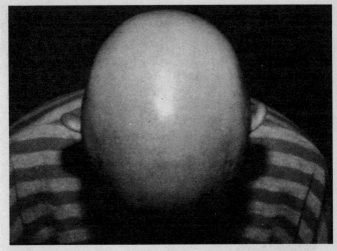

Photograph 12–2 (above) shows the same Dieter N. Kloss. We see the top of his head prior to daily application of *Thymu-Skin®*. Dieter will now begin to faithfully massage the shampoo and lotion into his head.

totalis et universalis. The senior author of their studies and jointly published papers was Dr. Moessler.

The current clinical investigation on Alopecia areata totalis and Alopecia areata universalis was undertaken because the product, GKL *Thymu-Skin®* Hair Treatment and Shampoo, had worked exceedingly well for previously investigated patients exhibiting symptoms of Alopecia areata and Alopecia androgenetica. Dr. Moessler had already published two additional medical papers about the success of this treatment in German journals of dermatology.[1,2]

Now, in an open clinical trial lasting up to twenty-four months on these twenty subjects, those who had been victimized by *alopecia areata totalis* and *alopecia areata universalis* were dispensed quantities of *Thymu-Skin®* for topical application. For 65 percent of the self-treating patients (twelve people), new hair growth at the scalp and/or on the

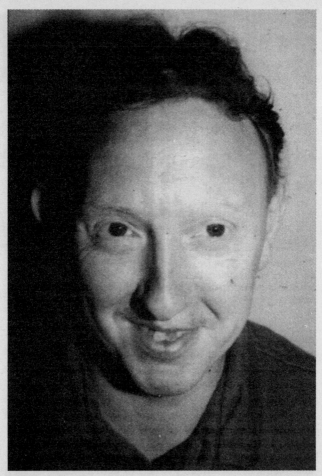

Photograph 12–3 (above) depicts Dieter N. Kloss nine months after he began the self-administered anti-baldness therapy with *Thymu-Skin®*. By the late spring of 1994 he has well-formed, tightly growing new head hair. He is also growing a beard, eyelashes, eyebrows, and hair on the rest of his body where he had none before.

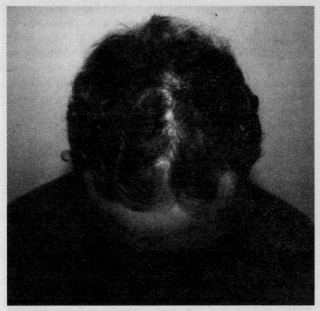

Photograph 12–4 (above) shows the patient nine months later; new hair growth is certainly apparent. The *Thymu-Skin®* Hair Treatment has taken hold as depicted by the clinic photographs furnished by dermatologist Klio Moessler, M.D., with the cooperation of her dermatology department chief, Professor Manfred Hagedorm, M.D.

body gradually occurred. In 40 percent of these same twelve hair-restored patients, a complete remission of their alopecia was achieved. Baldness went away within an average of sixteen months and has not returned in any form.

Evaluation of this Darmstadt study indicates that the complete alopecia remission rate in the *Thymu-Skin®* treated group was significantly greater than other medically established treatment regimens previously tried for patients. Prof. Dr. Hagedorn and Dr. Moessler wrote in their paper, ''A major advantage of the topically-applied *Thymu-Skin®* cosmetic was that its self-administration by the patients did not require frequent control examinations or weekly visits to any clinic.''[3]

Accompanying hair regrowth on the head within nine to twenty-four months of local therapy with *Thymu-Skin®*, complete hair regrowth on the body often simultaneously took place as well. This proves that the protomorphogenic effect of calf thymus extract was systemic and spread throughout the body from being absorbed into the patients' scalp.

The University of Heidelberg Gynecological Clinic Study

A fourth clinical study of *Thymu-Skin®* conducted in 1989 and lasting one year involves the German gynecologist/endocrinologist Professor Dr. med. Benno Runnebaum, Medical Director of The Department of Gynecology and Endocrinology at the University of Heidelberg in Heidelberg, Germany. Prof. Dr. med. Runnebaum had worked closely with Prof. Dr. med. Thomas Rabe, also of the Heidelberg women's clinic.

The title of Prof. Dr. med. Runnebaum's investigated thesis was "Topical Treatment of Diffuse Female Alopecia Using a Thymus-containing Preparation." Writing in his university-circulated medical paper, the professor stated:

A therapy formulation is incepted here for thymus extract, which contains a whole range of active substances as anabolic substances and nutrients for the cells. This present study is one of the first clinical test series in the application of hair shampoo or a hair treatment and is intended to document the proof of therapeutic success. . . . in twenty-two of twenty-nine female patients a measurable improvement occurred [for *alopecia diffusa*] after three to six months under conditions of consistent application. In this, the cooperation of the female patients was important in regard to the prescribed application and their dependableness in supervising the efficacy, which was done by counting of the hairs.

The female patients were selected after the [laboratory] tests in order to preclude the presence of dermatological or hormonal conditions or any deficiencies in their clinical pictures. Only thereafter was a monotherapy using *Thymu-Skin®* incepted. The decisive edge of *Thymu-Skin®* is its ability to effect cell regeneration and cell stabilization, while also applied directly as a topical agent. Through this method no side effects are found, and the product can be used by everybody without risk or the necessity of complicated directions.

During the evaluation of the data regarding the hair loss, a measurable improvement was found after three months of application: the daily hair loss fell from 203 hairs per day to 108 hairs per day. During a further checkup after six months, a median loss of eighty-five hairs per day was found. [Author's note: This is a normal fallout of hairs.]

Nine Scientific Studies of *Thymu-Skin®*

"My numerous clinical studies with several hundred patients confirm the effectiveness of *Thymu-Skin®* for hair growth in the treatment of alopecia areata and androgenetic alopecia," confirmed dermatologist Prof. Dr. med. M. Hagedorn in that third published paper from his clinic office at the Dermatological Department of the Municipal Hospital in Darmstadt, Germany. "In other studies with additional hundreds of patients, it has been effectively proven that hair loss can be stopped and hair growth reactivated if the roots are still intact. Clinical studies on patients who were losing hair caused by alopecia androgentica (pattern baldness) showed the *Thymu-Skin®* treatment was successful in 94 percent of the women and 67 percent of the men. Therapeutic success ratios increase with longer periods of treatment."[4]

The numerous clinical investigations mentioned by Dr. Hagedorn were conducted by nine scientific investigators in eight medical departments at eight locations in Germany and Austria. They were carried out by the following medical participants:

(1) oncological surgeon Prof. Dr. med. Helmuth Denck, M.D., in the Dept. of Surgery, Ludwig Boltzmann Institute for Clinical Oncology, Vienna City Hospital, Austria;

(2) dermatology clinic director Prof. Dr. med. Manfred Hagedorn, M.D., in the Municipal Clinics of Darmstadt, University of Frankfurt, Germany;

(3) the gynecological clinic honorary chairman Prof. Dr. med. Benno Runnebaum, M.D., at the Ruprecht-Karls University of Heidelberg, Germany;

(4) surgeon Dr. med. F. Preusser, M.D., in the Oncology/Surgery Dept. of the University Clinic of Muenster, Germany;

(5) hematologist Dr. med. H. Wilke, M.D., Dept. of Hematology/Oncology, the Medical University of Hannover Germany;

(6) medical statistician and information specialist Prof. Dr. Claus O. Koehler, Ph.D., in the Dept. of Medical and Biological Informatics, German Cancer Research Centre, Heidelberg Germany;

(7) surgical oncologist Prof. Dr. med. Ulrich Fink, M.D., in the Surgical Oncology Section, Dept. of Surgery, Surgical Clinic and Polyclinic of the Technical University of Munich, Germany;

(8) toxicologist/pharmacologist Prof. Dr. med. et Dr. pharm. Niels Peter Luepke, M.D., Chairman of the Division of Pharmacology and Toxicology, University of Osnabrueck, Germany;

(9) dermatologist Dr. Klio Moessler, M.D., at the Dermatology Clinic of the Municipal Clinics and Hospital of Darmstadt, Germany.

The Cytotoxic Hair Loss Study by Prof. Dr. Koehler

At the German Cancer Research Centre (DKFZ) in Heidelberg, Professor Dr. Claus O. Koehler, former Chief of the Department of Medical and Biological Informatics, had conducted an investigation on 251 cancer patients treated with cytotoxic agents. He used calf thymus extract combined with nutrients as the means of saving his clinic's patients from cytotoxic chemical baldness. It was mandatory that these subjects of Dr. Koehler's study undergo chemotherapy as the means to save their lives, at least temporarily.

The two cytotoxics used as treatment included 5-fluorouracil (5-Fu) for 144 patients and Adriamycin® for 107 patients. Chemotherapy had been administered because these people suffered with cancers involving either the stomach, lungs (bronchus and/or esophagus), kidneys, pancreas, or the lymphatic system (Hodgkin's disease).

For the 5-Fu-treated patients, no hair loss occurred for 68.5 percent of patients over age sixty and 58.9 percent under age sixty. For the Adriamycin-treated patients, hair was prevented from falling out in 48.4 percent of patients over age sixty and 10.6 percent under age sixty. The variance in percentages is partially due to 5-Fu being a less toxic drug than Adriamycin®.

Furthermore, younger people show a greater incidence of cell division than those older than sixty years. The hair follicles of a younger person would sooner fall to the destructive qualities of cytoxic agents than an older one whose mitosis ability had been slowed down by the buffeting of stressors during a longer life.

The type of cancer affecting a patient became a factor relating to hair loss, too. Some 89.7 percent of those patients affected with stomach carcinoma, in the judgment of oncologists, of necessity had to be treated with the more toxic Adriamycin®. Those patients diagnosed with breast cancer, colon cancer, and esophageal (broncheal) cancer most often received 5-Fu. The patients with breast and/or colon cancer usually kept their hair when topical *Thymu-Skin®* was used a week before or during chemotherapy.

Studying Alopecias Androgenetica and Areata

The Department of Dermatology of the Municipal Clinics at Darmstadt, Germany has also reported that calf thymus extract dispensed to patients as *Thymu-Skin®* provided great success against the two stubborn hair loss conditions, alopecia androgenetica and alopecia areata. This was a third study conducted by dermatologist Klio Moessler M.D., under the supervision of the clinic's dermatology department chairman Professor Manfred Hagedorn, M.D.

Alopecia androgenetica (also referred to as androgenetic alopecia) actually is genetically patterned baldness in men and women. Follicles in the scalp tend to stop producing hair at a certain time in life; although they continue their cycles of growth and rest. But the follicles' growth stage is becoming shorter and their resting longer. Also, each new hair produced is a little thinner and finer than the previous one. After some years, the follicles in a man's balding scalp can produce only fine, vellus "fuzz" that's nearly invisible to the naked eye. The follicles remain intact but incapable of growing a normal head of hair unless stimulated to do so with therapy such as calf thymus extract.[5]

For women, *alopecia androgenetica* presents a different pattern which leads only to a general thinning of hair on the top and sometimes on the sides of the scalp. Women rarely show bald spots on the crown and only occasionally have a receding front hairline. Typically, a woman will be around age sixty or seventy before reaching the full extent of her baldness, at which time her hair will also be finer and less luxuriant because of aging.[6] As Dr. med. Klio Moessler's study exhibits, this condition in women responds even more effectively to treatment with calf thymus extract than it does for men.

Alopecia areata is translated as meaning "patchy baldness,'' a condition that appears suddenly in people who have no apparent skin disorder or disease. It accounts for approximately 2 percent of all new patient visits to skin doctors in the United States and the United Kingdom. This type of patchy baldness is present in a family's history up to 9 percent of the time.

At the Churchill Hospital in Oxford, England, consulting dermatologist Rodney Dawber, M.A., M.B., Ch.B., and his textbook coauthor, Dominique Van Neste, M.D., Ph.D., Director of the Skin Study Center at Tournai, Belgium, declare Alopecia areata is a specific autoimmune disease. In their book, *Hair and Scalp Disorders,* they state: ''The strongest direct evidence for autoimmunity comes from the consistent findings of lymphocytic infiltrate in and around hair follicles and Langerhans cells have also been seen in the peribulbar region. . . . a reduction in the numbers of circulating T-cells occurs in Alopecia areata, the level of reduction being related to disease severity. Similarly, the impairment of helper T-cell function and the change in suppressor T-cell numbers may also reflect changes in disease activity.''[7]

Men and women both experience Alopecia areata, usually in the age groups between twenty and forty years. Since the cause has been unknown, it has been untreatable until now.[8] Dr. med. Klio Moessler has reported marvelous success by her dispensing calf thymus extract to patients at the Municipal Clinics of Darmstadt.

Therapeutic Successes Against Both Types of Alopecia

Dr. med. Moessler's results from her participating with Prof. Dr. med. Hagedorn in their third hair preservation and regrowth investigation were remarkable for changing the appearance of balding people. In her paper, she states:

Fifty-one patients with Alopecia androgenetica and sixteen patients with Alopecia areata were treated with

Thymu-Skin® (shampoo and tonic containing a thymus extract) over a period of twelve months. Sixty-seven percent of the male patients and 100 percent of the female patients with androgenetic alopecia had a benefit from this treatment. In 83 percent of the patients with Alopecia areata, *Thumu-Skin®* therapy resulted in partial or full regrowth of scalp hair. In female patients with Alopecia androgenetica the average daily hair loss [of individual hair strands] decreased from 139 (pretreatment) to 57 after twelve months. There was no remarkable change in male patients. In patients with Alopecia areata the average daily hair loss [individual hair strands] decreased from initially 245 to 10.

The two specific *Thymu-Skin®* products, hair shampoo and hair tonic manufactured by Thymu-Skin Cosmetic Klett-Loch GmbH of Mannheim, Germany, were utilized to acquire such marvelous results in Dr. Moessler's study. The gel, hair mask, and conditioner creme rinse were not used because they did not exist then. The therapeutic successes against both types of alopecia were analyzed in relation to the duration of hair loss for individual patients—both men and women. A scoring system was developed using the following classification: "Improvement' was +1, "no change" was 0 and "progression" [of hair loss] was-1. The duration of hair loss was classified in intervals of 1 to 12 months, 13 to 30 months, 31 to 60 months, and more than 60 months.

Thymu-Skin® Results for Male Pattern Baldness Are Good

Telling the story of success or failure for hair preservation are the detailed results of *Thymu-Skin®* usage shown below. They are divided into subjective improvement in relation to the duration of hair loss and objective therapeutic success evaluated by hair strand counts.

Subjective Improvement Relating to Duration of Hair Loss Among Men from Androgenetic Alopecia (Male Pattern Baldness)

- for men with male pattern baldness (MPB) present for from 1 to 12 months, 20 percent observed improvement (+1), 20 percent had no change (0), and 60 percent observed hair loss progression (-1);
- for men with MPB present for from 13 to 30 months, 50 percent (improvement (+1), 25 percent experienced no change (0), and 25 percent observed hair loss progression (-1);
- for men with MPB present for from 31 to 60 months, 25 percent had improvement (+1), 75 percent saw no change (0), none progressed to further hair loss (-1).

Objective Hair Strand Counts for Hair Preservation in Male Pattern Baldness

For men with MPB, the average number of daily hair strands lost by the male participants in this study was 119 before treatment, 98 after three months of treatment and only 76 after six months (less than the usual fallout of 80 strands per day).

Thymu-Skin® Results for Female Pattern Baldness Are Superior

For women with androgenetic alopecia the effects of using topically applied calf thymus extract containing nutrients were even better. As stated in her summary, Dr. Moessler said that 100 percent of her female patients benefited. Accordingly, she added an extra classification that described the impressions held by women in this study of *Thymu-Skin®* for the treatment of female pattern baldness (FPB).

Women's Subjective Impressions About Thymu-Skin® Usage for FPB

- For women with FPB, 49 percent had the impression that new hair growth was present after three months. They observed improvement (+1);
- For women with FPB, 51 percent saw no change (0) in three months of product usage;
- For women with FPB, 72 percent experienced good new hair growth-improvement (+1)—after six months of usage:
- For women with FPB, 21 percent saw no change (0) in six months;
- For women with FPB, 7 percent observed a progression of hair loss after six months of product use;
- For women with FPB, 67 percent observed much improvement (+1) after nine months of self-administering *Thymu-Skin®;*
- For women with FPB, 19 percent observed no change (0) after nine months;
- For women with FPB, 14 percent felt that hair loss progression (-1) had occurred.

At the conclusion of this study, all of the participating women stated their personal satisfaction with the therapeutic success they experienced in treating androgenetic alopecia. Their hair loss either stopped or they saw new hair growth with which they were highly pleased.

Subjective Improvement Relating to Duration of Hair Loss Among Women from Androgenetic Alopecia (Female Pattern Baldness)

- for women with female pattern baldness (FPB) present for from 1 to 12 months, 83 percent observed improvement (+1), 17 percent had no change (0), and none of the women observed further hair loss progression (-1);

- for women with FPB present for from 13 to 30 months, 78 percent had improvement (+1), 22 percent experienced no change (0), and none observed any progression (-1) to further hair loss;
- for women with FPB present for from 31 to 60 months, 60 percent had improvement (+1), 22 percent saw no change (0), and, surprisingly, 18 percent reported they had progressed to further hair loss (-1).

Objective Hair Strand Counts for Hair Preservation in Female Pattern Baldness

For women with FPB, the average number of daily hair strands lost by the female participants in this study was 139 before treatment with the calf thymus extract, 90 after three months of treatment, 80 after six months, and 57 after twelve months (less than the usual female hair fallout).

Subjective Improvement Relating to Duration of Hair Loss from Alopecia Areata (AA) Among Both Sexes

- for study participants having AA present for from 1 to 12 months, 40 percent observed improvement (+1), 40 percent had no change (0), and 20 percent observed hair loss progression (-1);
- for subjects with AA present for from 13 to 30 months, 50 percent had improvement (+1), 50 percent experienced no change (0), and none observed hair loss progression (-1);
- for patients having AA present for from 31 to 60 months, 60 percent had improvement (+1), 40 percent saw no change (0), and none progressed to further hair loss (-1).

For all patients with a duration of hair loss of more than 60 months, new hair growth was observed where there had been bare scalp patches before.

Objective Hair Strand Counts for Hair Preservation in Alopecia Areata

For men and women having AA, the average number of daily hair strands lost by the participants in this study was 245 before treatment with the shampoo and tonic of *Thymu-Skin®*, 195 after three months of treatment, 164 after six months, 80 after nine months, and only 10 after twelve months.

During the total period of treatment, *Thymu-Skin®* showed no local or systemic adverse side effects, except that T-lymphocyte counts improved somewhat, which was a positive immune system response.

Subjective Impressions About Thymu-Skin® Usage for Alopecia Areata (AA)

- For men and women participants in this study who had AA, 31 percent had the impression that new hair growth was present after three months. They observed improvement (+1);
- 44 percent saw no change (0) in three months of product usage;
- 25 percent observed a progression toward more hair loss;
- 47 percent experienced good new hair growth—an improvement (+1)—after six months of usage;
- 33 percent saw no change (0) in six months;
- 20 percent observed a progression of hair loss after six months of product use;
- 75 percent observed much improvment (+1) after nine months of self-administering *Thymu-Skin®;*
- 17 percent observed no change (0) after nine months;
- 8 percent felt that hair loss progression (-1) had occurred;
- After twelve months of local therapy with *Thymu-Skin®* there was no progression toward further hair loss, but rather improvment in 86 percent of patients with alopecia areata. In 14 percent the status of their hair growth did not change.

CHAPTER THIRTEEN

The Hair-Preserving Properties of *Thymu-Skin*®

The chief sales executive for a pharmaceutical company in Atlanta, Georgia, dynamic thirty-two-year-old Theresa Ann Klein, was conscious of her appearance as she presented it to health practitioners. To introduce new drugs to the medical profession, she visited clinics, hospitals, and doctors' offices as part of her job. How she looked to others, therefore, was important to the success of her sales effort. Yet, when her handsome husband, Arthur, suggested that she should start using a hair-preserving product, the woman's reaction to his comment was "you're out of your mind!

"But the truth that I admit only to myself is that Arthur was probably correct. In all honesty, my hair had definitely been getting thinner. I was finding too many clumps and loose hairs stuck on my comb and in the bristles of my brush," Theresa told me, "but didn't everybody?

"Still, I thought about the progress my husband had made with his receding hairline. Arthur had been balding for many years, but now he was achieving good results by his daily use of a line of imported hair-preserving products called *Thymu-Skin*®. So after a while I decided to give his same Shampoo and Hair-Treatment Lotion a try for a couple of months. Then, some weeks into using these two items, I added the other three *Thymu-Skin*® products, the Conditioner Creme Rinse, the Hair-Treatment Mask, and the Hair-

Treatment Gel,'' Theresa explained. ''I did this because thickening of my hair became much greater than I had expected. The *Thymu-Skin®* was working.

''After I had shampooed and applied the lotion only twice, my hair loss seemed to decrease noticeably. In fact, my husband even accused me of picking up fallen hair strands off the bathroom sink where they used to accumulate,'' she states. ''Such a situation was encouraging because all my life my hair had been thin, lifeless, boring, and coming out in patches. But now I noticed a certain sheen and body developing. There had been a time when I tried everything I could find that promised to thicken my hair, but each item always ended in my disappointment. The products' exaggerated claims caused me to lose faith in all of them.

''Now, almost half-year a year has gone by since I began in earnest to apply the five *Thymu-Skin®* hair products, and I love what they are doing for me,'' Theresa says. ''Everyone who sees me offers compliments on my looks. And the doctors are ordering more pharmaceuticals than ever from my company.

''When recently I visited my local beauty salon for a hair shaping, the stylist praised me enthusiastically on my hair's new sturdy texture, full-bodied thickness, and dazzling shine. She remembered when it had been dull, fragile, and full of broken ends. Most often separate hair strands were falling down around my shoulders and onto clothing,'' says Theresa. ''But, all of that has changed for the better now that I routinely apply *Thymu-Skin®* Shampoo, Conditioner, Hair Mask, Gel, and especially the Hair-Treatment Lotion. I'll never use any other hair preparation again. I have to admit that my husband was right, and I owe Arthur an apology for how I had snapped at him six months ago.''

Dermatology Today Announces the Advent of *Thymu-Skin®*

With banner headlines, the May 1992 issue of *Dermatology Today (Dermatologie Heute),* published in Berlin for the information of skin and hair specialists attending the 37th Continuing Education Seminar of the Professional Association of German Dermatologists, announced:

"There is now reliable proof of hair-preserving properties available from specially prepared thymus extract called *Thymu-Skin*® on different forms of baldness which one encounters in medical practice. Even in cases of alopecia areata, alopecia androgenetica (male and female pattern baldness), and telogen alopecia (diffuse hair loss), when hair follicles stay intact hair strands can be made to regrow."[1]

This monthly newspaper circulated to German-speaking dermatologists all over Europe went on to report on the Darmstadt Municipal Clinic study conducted by Dr. med. Klio Moessler and Prof. Dr. med. Manfred Hagedorn (discussed at the end of Chapter Twelve.)

Two years before the dermatology seminar was held, another German consumer newspaper. *The New Leaf (Das Neue Blatt),* reported in a weekly summer issue. " 'People who usually swim in the ocean or a swimming pool have to take care of their hair more often. Salt water and chlorine dry out the scalp especially in combination with sun and wind,' warns oncological surgery professor Dr. med. Helmuth Denck [of Vienna, Austria]. 'Itchiness, formation of dandruff, increased hair loss, or even inflammation are the result.' Professor Denck advises all persons to use *Thymu-Skin*® for hair protection. This remedy is known to be especially effective after what the now concluded clinical studies at the Heidelberg University Women's Clinic have shown about the benefits of using this hair strengthening preparation. The University's results are based on all kinds of hair loss."[2]

Relief of Dandruff from Using *Thymu-Skin*®

As indicated additionally by Prof. Dr. med. Denck, *Thymu-Skin*® counteracts dandruff. Although it is present in at least 25 percent of the world's population, flaking of the scalp in the form of dandruff is not a normal condition. Dandruff may be referred to by some dermatologists as *seborrhea*. In that case it is caused by abnormal regulation of the sebaceous glands and is characterized by an excessive production of sebum, the semifluid secretion of these glands. The dandruff patient complains of excessively greasy and unmanageable hair that not only fails to be helped by shampooing but actually becomes worsened by it. Flaking with acute or chonic inflammation of the scalp is called *seborrheic dermatitis*.[3]

Dr. med. Klio Moessler tends to disagree with those dermatologists who consider drandruff a form of seborrhea. Dr. Moessler advises, "Dandruff is similar to scaling of the skin. Seborrhea is excessive sebum production. Dandruff is often combined or caused by seborrhea. And dandruff plus seborrhea plus inflammation is seborrheic dermatitis."

In contrast with ordinary shampoos, *Thymu-Skin®* Shampoo applied to an oily scalp which is flaking dandruff works exceedingly well to stop such flaking. The shampoo and its accompanying hair lotion must be applied every day for four weeks and thereafter every second day. When the scalp's condition normalizes, dandruff disappears altogether. After that, the hair may be shampooed with *Thymu-Skin®* merely twice a week. (Note each time one shampoos, the *Thymu-Skin®* Hair Treatment Lotion should be used directly afterward to assure dandruff stays away.)

Prof. Dr. med. Thomas Rabe, Associate Professor of Obstetrics and Gynecology in the Division of Gynecological Endocrinology at the University Women's Hospital in Heidelberg, reports, "*Thymu-Skin®* is efficacious against the different forms of alopecia in men and women, and it also works for children who have Alopecia areata. It doesn't cause side effects and therefore can be used long-term and for permanent application for patients with Alopecia androgenetica (also known as Alopecia hereditaria). The latter is a disease which can be influenced into producing new hair growth but not cured. Still, one can apply the products of *Thymu-Skin®* forever. For myself, I readily would use *Thymu-Skin®* in the case of hair loss."

A Possible Mode of Action for *Thymu-Skin®*

Since the exact working mechanism of this biologically active calf thymus extract is hypothesized but not entirely known, researchers clinically dispensing the hair-protective product have made a few calculated assumptions. The doctors believe that dysfunctional miniature hair follicles become altered at the site of their terminals. There is a really different possible mode of action for *Thymu-Skin®*.

Out of an increased efficiency of the patient's immune system from absorption of the thymus extract through the skin of the scalp, the follicles are stimulated to give rise to tiny new hairs, which eventually will grow into terminal (long, thick, pigmented) hairs. The follicles become excited into functioning again. In particular this possible mode of action may be true for those patients taking cytotoxic treatment for overcoming cancer or other degenerative diseases.

Although the information has not been published in the medical literature, it's suspected by German gynecologists and dermatologists that the restoration of physiological homeostasis additionally occurs from *Thymu-Skin®* application for those various overactive components of the immune system which tend to produce minor, local, autoimmune attacks of the hair follicles. Such responses of self against self potentially being neutralized, hair loss diminishes or ceases altogether. The mechanism of autoimmune attack becomes neutralized by the calming effect of the hair preservation formula.

The main active agents of any *Thymu-Skin®* product are short-chained peptides (labeled chemically for identification by the manufacturer as *GKL 01*). These tiny peptides are formulated in connection with vitamin and mineral nutrients, enzymes, and free amino acids. All of them become intermixed with the peptide extract taken from the calf thymus gland. The peptides are highly penetrating into the integument of the scalp and carry the nutrients, enzymes, and amino acids with themselves.

How the Hair Preparation Formula Is Made

The thymus glands are taken from calves already slaughtered for veal cutlets and chops. The calves chosen are never older than six months and come from American livestock (not European) absolutely free of antibiotics, steroids or other drugs potentially harmful to human beings. The peptides are delivered as a specially prepared thymus extract. Particular amino acids intermixed with the extract are methionine and cystine, for they have an affinity to nourishing hair follicles. (See Chapter Fourteen for a full listing of the additional nutrient content of the hair preparation formula.)

The thymus glands are autoclaved according to standards set by the World Health Organization at a temperature of 136°C and an elevated barometric pressure for a minimum of 60 minutes. The thymus extract obtained goes on to undergo a proprietary procedure that opens up the protein peptides so as to exclude any incubations of those certain destructed proteins called *Prions*. The hydrolisate thus formed is clear of bacteria, viruses, fungi, protozoa, parasites, and any other pathological microorganisms. The thymus is then pulverized in a sterile environment resulting in a 100 percent water-soluble extract. Supervisory analysis is performed with every batch by the independent research institute, Orpegen Pharma GmbH of Heidelberg, Germany.

The subsequent thymus hydrolysate extract consisting of a combination of short-chained peptides with free amino acids, vitamins, minerals, and enzymes are then tested and retested against the five most common, conventionally known extracts offered in the biological marketplace. The object of such testing is to confirm that *Thymu-Skin®* peptides possess maximum biological and immunological activity. With positive peptide activity response at its optimum, this peptide ingredient is labeled the *Thymus GKL 01* agent. It is of the highest pharmaceutical-grade quality and corresponding safety data sheets containing analytical data are kept.

Toxicity checking for thymus extract *GKL 01* is unnecessary, as throughout Europe thymus is acknowledged as a food. It is offered in all well-reputed restaurants as a tasty dish—a delicacy—called *sweetbreads*. Lacking adverse side effects, thymus extracts are readily allowed for use in cosmetics. Although *Thymu-Skin®* brings about a therapeutic effect just like a drug, its ingredients allow this hair-preserving product to be classified by the United States and German Food and Drug Administrations as a cosmetic.

All countries in which *Thymu-Skin®* has been introduced as a commercial product have had their ethics associations examine it. Because the preparation has been subjected to no unusual or extra restricting regulations, invariably it is classified as "unobjectionable." Humans suffering from hair loss who are recruited from university hospitals, medical schools, and academic teaching hospitals have participated in numerous double-blind, placebo-controlled clinical trials. Most are patients who have been referred by their own dermatologists, internists, gynecologists, and other health professionals. The study participants are referred because they have failed to find viable hair growth therapy from the use of drugs already available on the market. These balding patients are the most difficult type to treat, but they do well with this hair preparation.

Biological and Immunological Activity of *GKL 01 AND GKL 02*

In order to manufacture *GKL 01* as a synthetic product having a closely natural identity and then to register it with the German Health Authority (Germany's food and drug administration) popularly known to the public and to health professionals as *B farm* (previously called *Bundesgesundheitamt* or BGA), Thymu-Skin Cosmetic, a division of Klett-Loch GmbH of Mannheim, sponsored a series of experiments and other laboratory investigations. They were undertaken for four years by Orpegen Pharma GmbH. Observed in the test tube *(in vitro)* and later in animals *(in vivo*), the peptides of *GKL 01* caused a rapid increase of T-lymphocytes. The same thing happens in humans when the peptides are applied to their bald heads; the people show an immunological enhancement effect. Thus, coating the scalp with any of the *Thymu-Skin®* products simultaneously offers two advantages: (a) it stimulates hair follicles to grow hair and (b) it improves the activity of one's immune system.

Despite the hair-preserving product line being classified in Germany as a cosmetic, that country's national health insurance plan (similar to Medicare in the United States) reimburses cancer patients when they use *Thymu-Skin®*. Oncologists prescribe it. Also, some German private insurance carriers are reimbursing users who file claims stating that they have "diseased hair loss". Thymus gland extract from calf is the market leader against baldness in most German-speaking countries.

Germany's *B Farm* checks the product's manufacturing process continuously, and now the agency has allowed *GKL 01* to be made as a synthetic. These new short-chained, synthetic peptides (identified in the laboratory with the label *Synthetic Thymus Peptide Library* or STPI) are far superior therapeutically than natural peptides derived from the original source, calf thymus gland. STPI are nature-identical but standardized and guaranteed to always have the same unchanged quality of substance. As pulverized material, synthetic peptides are exceedingly soluble in water at temperatures between 20°C and 21°C, and this property allows them to be absorbed well into the scalp. When sold commercially, the synthetic STPI will be re-identified as *GKL 02* in contrast to the natural peptides labeled *GKL 01*.

Both *GKL 01* and *GKL 02* show up as immunologically active, and they afford a great amount of hair follicle growth stimulation. But *GKL 02* is more stimulative. An enhanced hair preservation effect takes place for any person rubbing these peptides into the scalp because the immunological system becomes invigorated. Also there is a docking-on of the male hormones (androgens) to hair follicle receptor cells so that hair strands can grow without hindrance.

To prove that this increased short-chained peptide biological activity occurs in human subjects, two placebo-controlled, randomized double-blind trials are underway now. The clinical studies have gone into their second year of investigation and will be reported sometime after the publication of this book.

CHAPTER FOURTEEN

Results That May Be Expected from Using *Thymu-Skin®*

There are five different *Thymu-Skin®* hair products that preserve hair follicles and/or stimulate dormant but live follicles into regrowth. A consumer may choose to begin with only two products.

How to Use the Formulations

Being the two items investigated during clinical studies done in Germany, the **Thymu-Skin®** Shampoo and **Thymu-Skin®** Hair Treatment Lotion are the really important formulations to use. The fundamental principle of the shampoo is to cleanse the scalp with tiny penetrating thymus peptides. Since these peptides are broken down into an extremely small length—only 300 angstroms—they diffuse themselves into the hair follicles better than any other mode of cleanser. They clean out each follicle of accumulated oil, dirt, debris, and other waste and prepare the scalp for receiving a dose of the treatment lotion.

These two products—shampoo and hair treatment lotion—work synergistically, and they are packaged together in kits—small and large. The small kit contains one bottle of 100 milliliters (ml) of shampoo and one bottle of 100 ml of the treatment lotion. (A milliliter is one thousandth of a liter, and one liter is 33.814 ounces or roughly, one oz. contains 30 ml., and there are 30 drops in one ml.) Each of the small-size kit products will last six to eight weeks, depending on the volume of hair to which they are applied. A larger area of scalp that is thinning or balding actually uses less liquid than hairy areas because the solutions are more readily spread across the scalp's smooth skin.

The larger *Thymu-Skin*® hair preservation kit contains one 200 ml. bottle of shampoo and one 200 ml. bottle of hair treatment lotion. Each lasts approximately three to four months, again depending on the volume of hair and the areas of thinning or balding.

The usual experience of users is that large amounts of hair fallout around the sink or in the shower diminish steadily. The user notices a decrease of hair fall within the first week of only using the shampoo. If the user has observed balding or thinning of head hair for less than five years, he or she is likely to notice new hair growth as early as two to three months. Because it lasts twice as long as the small size, the larger-size kit is a better value. If hair loss has been occurring for longer than five years, it could take anywhere from twelve to eighteen months to see new hair growth. Usually after eighteen months, if the *Thymu-Skin*® combination of ingredients hasn't helped, the hair follicles on remaining bald areas are probably dead and nothing applied will help to restore them to life.

The *Thymu-Skin*® **Hair Treatment Gel** is a higher concentration of thymus peptides, vitamins, minerals, enzymes, and amino acids. It was developed to be used in conjunction with the shampoo and treatment lotion. The gel is a kind of ''miracle grow'' that tends to produce follicular stimulation more quickly. Because it's so very concentrated, only place the gel onto the balding or thinning areas for intervals of twelve hours, and use it separately from the shampoo and lotion. One might apply the gel in the evening and go to sleep with it spread over the scalp; then in the morning shampoo it away and put on the lotion for wearing during the balance of the day.

The *Thymu-Skin*® **Hair Treatment Mask** is more of a

setting lotion. It is prepared as a gelled type of substance that one applies to towel-dried hair after the shampoo and hair treatment lotion have been used. The hair mask is placed on the head between the hairs and combed through so that these hairs become covered with a protective coating. This coating holds off ultraviolet rays, X-rays, cosmic rays, and other adverse environmental influences from affecting new hair growth. Balding airline personnel who fly as part of their occupation would benefit greatly from usage of the hair treatment mask. Also it makes the hair feel healthy to the touch and look shiny.

The *Thymu-Skin®* **Conditioner Creme Rinse** is some-what more expensive than other hair rinses, but it makes the hair strands very soft and silky to the touch. This texture holds in place for an extra long period. The conditioner contains the thymus peptides and avocado oils which help to regulate the fat metabolism of the scalp. It may be left in place to condition for up to fifteen minutes (with a towel wrapped around the head) twice a week without any worry of clogging the hair follicles.

If someone wishes to condition the hair with something other than the *Thymu-Skin®* Conditioner Creme Rinse, use a natural cosmetic product and only put it on the hair ends. Otherwise, if this substitute conditioner is allowed to coat the scalp, it will undo the *Thymu-Skin®* Shampoo's cleansing of the scalp and its hair follicles.

As for other shampoos, they may posses peptides which break down to the usual, larger size of 500 angstroms. These bigger peptides won't penetrate the scalp to clean out the hair follicles. Clogging from debris then develops.

Permanent waves, dyeing, and highlighting the hair have no adverse effect on the success of *Thymu-Skin®*. However, it's recommended that only high-quality brand products be used for these purposes. Afterward, neutralize possible abuse of the hair follicles by reapplying the *Thymu-Skin®* Conditioner Creme Rinse and Hair Treatment Mask.

Using a hair dryer is not recommended for managing the hair, as it causes the scalp to perspire, become dehydrated, and undergo deprivation of necessary minerals, resulting in skin dryness, itching, dandruff, and hair loss. If a hair dryer must be used, consider following these practices:

- Hold the hot air blowing apparatus to one side of the head and direct it from below in an upward direction and away from the scalp.
- Insure that no hot air reaches the scalp directly.
- After applying hair treatment lotion, under no circumstances use a hair dryer or the lotion will be dissipated into the air as an evaporant. One's effort and investment will then be lost.

How Often to Apply the Hair Treatment

To insure new hair growth or to prevent any further receding hairline, *Thymu-Skin*® Hair Treatment should be applied to the scalp twice a day for four weeks. Thereafter it can be put on once a day for six to eighteen months, depending on the severity of hair loss. After one's baldness is decreased and hair growth is more predominant, usage can first be reduced to every second day and then to twice a week. When the *Thymu-Skin*® Hair Treatment Revitalizer is applied to the scalp, a brisk one-minute massage should be administered each time. Additionally, wash the hair at least twice a week with *Thymu-Skin*® Shampoo. This is excellent naturally-exciting therapy for the hair follicles of people who have been victims of one or more of four particular scalp problems: female or male patterned baldness, *alopecia medicamentosa* (chemotherapy), a*lopecia totalis,* and *alopecia universalis.*

Only those regions on the scalp containing enough live hair follicles will show good hair growth. If patches of the scalp hold dead follicles, no hair will rise from them. Usually hair preservation and even new hair growth will happen for people who are still in the process of losing their hair. For those who had experienced a sudden baldness occurring from allergy, deficiency, menopause, pregnancy, metallic toxicity, or another reason associated with pathology, the health problem is best corrected first. Then, without question, *Thymu-Skin®* does the job exceedingly well. If this product is applied one week before and during mild or moderate chemotherapy, there won't be any hair loss for the patient. Such a fact is verified by numbers of German oncologists.

Keep in mind that *Thymu-Skin®* is a doctor-recommended cosmetic product sold without prescription, over-the-counter, and for self-administration.

For longstanding baldies like me, in which male pattern baldness is an inherited trait *(alopecia hereditaria),* there is no hope of much hair restoration. Even so, Dr. Moessler told me, "If somebody has members of his or her family who are bald, and he or she does not want to be bald as well, he or she should use *Thymus-Skin®* as a preventative, starting at a young age and continuing for a long period."

Acting on Dr. Moessler's advice—absolutely believing in her expertise—I have prevailed upon my thirty-three-year-old son, Jules Louis Walker of San Francisco, California, to apply the *Thymu-Skin®* products to his head. Jules told me that he is observing some additional retention of his hair with less fallout. Visiting with him recently, I can affirm that hair on his head is remaining in place. While Jules is not regrowing any big beautiful mane he's not getting any balder either.

As for me, even with being age sixty-eight, I studiously apply the lotion and shampoo once daily. And you know what? After a couple of years of usage, my wife says that she sees new hairs sprouting from various areas of my scalp where follicles apparently still remain alive. There aren't many of them, but some hairs are three inches long. They've been awakened from their state of slumber by my faithfully using the *Thymu-Skin®* Shampoo and *Thymu-Skin®* Hair Treatment lotion.

In doing so, it's a fact that Jules, all other users of *Thymu-Skin®* and I are providing good health for ourselves. Through the scalp, we are feeding our immune systems a broad spectrum of nutrients—those very healthy ingredients comprising the *Thymu-Skin®* formula. In association with the highly penetrating small-chained peptides, they are carried into the bloodstream and travel around to the rest of the body. The combination preparations are stimulating the growth of hair and, optionally, the growth of skin and nails, as well as for preventing and eliminating the loss of hair. Through the skin of the scalp, the following nutrients, under U.S. Patent PCT/DE95/01745, are nourishing the total physiology, most especially hair follicles, epidermis, and nails:

Provitamin A (beta carotene)	Methionine
Vitamin B_1 (thiamin)	Cystine
Vitamin B_2 (riboflavin)	Flax oil
Pantothenic acid	Lactalbumin
Biotin	Calcium
Folic acid (folate)	Glycerol
Nicotinamide	Vegetable oils
Vitamin B_6 (pyridoxine)	CoEnzyme Q_{10} (ubiquinone)
Vitamin B_{12} (cyanocobalamine)	Stabilizer E 420
Vitamin C (ascorbic acid)	Selenium
Vitamin E (D,L alpha tocopherol)	Calf thymus extract

Results That May Be Expected from Using Calf Thymus Products

A person may or may not expect excellent results from using the newly developed *Thymu-Skin®* hair products. One's expectation may be modified in accordance with four prevailing factors:

(A) heredity as a source of androgen excess,
(B) how long one has been bald,

(C) alopecia related to androgenic pattern hair loss,
(D) loss of hair from advanced age.

If baldness is genetic (factor A), there's not much to be done.

If baldness has been present for a couple of decades (factor B), chances of hair regrowth are lessened considerably. On bald spots which are more than four years old, the thymus extract hair treatment does not result in new growth, because the hair roots usually have already been rejected by the scalp. In the case of thinning hair, new hair growth may fill in the sparse area and thicken further. This is because *Thymu-Skin®* reactivates inactive hair roots which are still intact, at the same time improving the blood flow to the scalp.

If male pattern baldness (MPB) or female pattern baldness (FPB) is the predominant difficulty (factor C), the rate of success may increase considerably (see Chapter Twelve). Women especially experience beneficial responses of their FPB when the thymus preparation is employed. (Dr. med. Moessler reports that it's 100 percent.) MPB doesn't seem to react to applications of *Thymu-Skin®* quite as well. (The Darmstadt Municipal Clinics dermatologist says it's 67 percent.)

If over age sixty-five (factor D), don't expect a lot of hair to grow; however, some will make its appearance if any live follicles are left.

Until now, there has been no therapy that's been successful in regrowing permanent hair that is lost due to male pattern baldness. Androgen causes the hair bulb to shrink and cuts off blood supply to the bulb, making it impossible for that bulb to produce new hair. Instead, vellus hairs, those wispy, almost invisible short hairs often seen on infants' heads, get substituted for colored terminal hair on the scalp. That's not good for an older adult's potential hair regrowth. Vellus hair can never be reawakened into normal terminal hair.

Still, the Dermatology Department of the Municipal Clinics of Darmstadt in Germany has had good success with overcoming male and female patterned baldness, especially in women. Prof. Dr. Hagedorn and Dr. Klio Moessler have edited this book's original manuscript with the admonition that if a young man or woman who is experiencing hair loss will begin using *Thymu-Skin®* early enough, baldness can be avoided because original hair growth can be retained. Therefore, I am authorized to say that if anyone is victimized by *alopecia totalis, alopecia universalis, alopecia adrogenetica, telogen alopecia* (diffuse baldness), or faces the potential of *alopecia medicamentosa* from toxic drug ingestion, a good hair growing result can be expected from using the five *Thymu-Skin®* hair-preserving products.

Ingredients in the *Thymu-Skin®* hair formula have a broad range of application for the prevention of hair loss and the regrowth of fallen hair. The positive effects of this hair preserver in gel, conditioner, hair mask, lotion and shampoo forms are for the following purposes:

- to use on a prophylactic basis for the avoidance of hair loss
- to reduce moderate and heavy hair loss
- to diminish hair thinning during menopause
- to prevent hair loss during cancer chemotherapy
- to quickly restore hair growth following chemotherapy
- to stop dandruff formation following hormonal treatment
- to relieve generalized dandruff and itching scalp
- to stimulate new hair growth if the hair roots are still intact
- to replace weak hair strands with strong hair

Thymu-Skin® physiologically accomplishes regrowth of hair as a result of the synergistic effects of its numerous nutritional ingredients; yet, an individual's consistent and correct application of the product line is absolutely essential for a high rate of success. After approximately four weeks of product usage, a reduction in hair fallout may be expected. Hair growth stabilizes, and the separate hair strands exhibit their natural shine besides becoming stronger. People with pale yellow hair or those troubled by matted hair or split hair strands will particularly notice their hair roots, shafts, and follicles showing positive reactions. Also itching scalp, dandruff, and slight to moderate hair loss will be much relieved or cease altogether within four to eight weeks of self-treatment.

At least six to eighteen months of treatment with *Thymu-Skin®* are required in order to achieve a complete normalization of hair growth. If hair loss has been heavy and present for more than four years, don't expect new and stronger hair growth until up to eighteen months of application have passed.

If *Thymu-Skin®* treatment is discontinued after improvement has been noted, a relapse after several months might happen. In order to assure maintenance of the success of the therapy, it's recommended that *Thymu-Skin®* usage be continued indefinitely a couple of times per week. But such continuing procedure isn't mandatory, and an individual has every reason to experiment with his or her own hair regrowth.

Good luck with *your* hair restoration!

APPENDIX ONE

Sources of Products Cited in This Book

Pegasus Ginsenocides processed from North American ginseng are distributed throughout North America by **Pegasus USA,** Post Office Box 6553, Metairie, Louisiana 70009; telephone (888) 259-9036 or (504) 834-3645; teleFAX (504) 828-8583; E-mail address: pegasususa@mindspring.com.

Haelan 951™ is imported into the United States and distributed throughout North America and to other parts of the world by **Haelan Products, Inc.,** 18568 142nd Avenue Northeast, Building F, Woodinville, Washington 98072; telephone (800) 542-3526, or (425) 482-2645; teleFAX (800) 258-2173.

Thymu-Skin® in all its varieties of form, Shampoo, Hair Treatment Revitalizer, Conditioner Creme Rinse, Gel, and Hair Mask, are imported from Mannheim, Germany and distributed throughout North America and to some other parts of the world by **ThymuSkin USA,** located at P.O. Box 931104, Norcross, Georgia 30003; telephone (800) 214-8631 or (770) 935-9104; teleFAX (770) 935-0351; website: www.biotekusa.com.

APPENDIX TWO

Footnoted References

Preface

1. Clarke, Thurston. *Equator: A Journey.* (New York: William Morrow, 1988).

2. Clarke, Thurston. "Going, going, gone." *The New York Times Magazine* Sept. 9, 1990, p. 82.

3. *Encyclopedia Americana, International Edition* (New York: Americana Corporation, 1966), Volume 12, pp. 613 & 614.

4. Sadick, N.S.; Richardson, D.C. *Your Hair: Helping to Keep It.* (Yonkers, New York: Consumer Reports Books, 1992), p. 1.

5. Dawber, R. and Van Neste, D. *Hair and Scalp Disorders: Common Presenting Signs, Differential Diagnosis and Treatment.* (Philadelphia: J.B. Lippincott Co., 1995), p. 245.

6. Thompson, W. and Shapiro, J. *Alopecia Areata: Understanding and Coping with Hair Loss.* (Baltimore: The Johns Hopkins University Press, 1996), p. 12.

7. Jacobs, S. *The Big Fall.* (Burnaby, BC, Canada: New Century Books, 1992), p. 23.

Introduction

1. Hoffer, A. and Walker, M. *Putting It All Together: The New Orthomolecular Nutrition.* (New Canaan, Connecticut: Keats Publishing, Inc., 1996).

2. Hoffer, A. and Walker, M . *Smart Nutrients: A Guide to Nutrients that Can Prevent and Reverse Senility.* (Garden City Park, New York: Avery Publishing Group, Inc., 1994), p. 54.

3. Fleming, R. and Mayer, T. *The Everyman's Guide to Hair Replacement.* (Austin, Texas: EquiMedia Corporation, 1994), pp. 75 & 76.

4. Sadick, N.S. and Richardson, D.C. *Your Hair: Helping to Keep It.* (Yonkers, New York: Consumer Reports Books, 1992). pp. 61–64.

5. Rutz, D. and Geraci, R. "Don't get scalped." *Men's Health* 12(6):82–83, July/August 1997.

Chapter One
Psychological Aspects of Losing Your Hair

1. Aldhizer, T. Gerald; Krop, Thomas M.; and Dunn, Joseph W. *The Doctor's Book on Hair Loss* (Englewood Cliffs, New Jersey: Prentice Hall, 1983), pp. 5–14.

2. Picardie, R. "This is Tracy Quinn, who began to go bald at 12, a misfortune most women could not endure, including those who mimic it." *The Independent* 3211 :S10 (1 page), October 8, 1996.

3. "Hair loss in women: it's more common than you may think." *Mayo Clinic Health Letter* 15(2):4 (2 pages), February 1997.

4. Rapaport, J. and Rubin, B.M. "Are you losing your hair?" *Good Housekeeping* 225 (1):41 (3 pages), July 1997.

5. Renken, K. "Losing my mind over losing my hair." *Cosmopolitan* January 1993, p. 84.

6. Marin, R. "Kiss it good-bye." *Gentlemen's Quarterly* August 1992, pp. 172—177.

7. *America On-Line* August, 1996.

8. Cash, T.F. "The psychological effects of androgenetic

alopecia in men." *Journal of the American Academy of Dermatology* 26(6):926–931, June 1992.

9. Cash, T.F. "Psychological effects of androgenetic alopecia among women: comparisons with female controls and with balding men. A technical report to The Upjohn Company," Kalamazoo, Michigan, August 1991.

10. Chiarapa, M. and Harris, L.C. "I went bald at 33." *Ladies Home Journal* 113(6):36 (3 pages), June 1996.

Chapter Two
What Baldness Is and Why It Develops

1. "Hair—the long and the short of it." *Science News* December 24 & 31, 1994, p. 427.

2. Dauber, R. and Van Neste, D. *Hair and Scalp Disorders: Common Presenting Signs, Differential Diagnosis and Treatment* (Philadelphia: J.B. Lippincott Company, 1995), p. 96.

3. Solamon, T. "Genetic factors in male alopecia. In Baccaredda-Bov, A.; Maretti, G .K..; and Frey, F.R. (eds.): *Biopathology of Pattern Alopecias* (Baser, Switzerland: S. Karger, 1968), pp. 39–49.

4. Ebling, F.J. "The hair cycle and its regulation." *Clinical Dermatology* 6:67-73, 1988.

5. Schmidt, J.B. "Nuclear and cytosol androgen receptors in androgen-dependent dermatoses in female patients." *Experimental Clinical Endocrinology* 90:107–112, 1987.

6. Olsen, Elise A. *Disorders of Hair Growth: Diagnosis and Treatment.* (New York: McGraw-Hill, Inc., 1994).

7. Moschella, S. L. and Hurley, H.J. *Dermatology, Third edition* (Philadelphia: W.B. Saunders Co., 1992), pp. 1541–1560.

Chapter Three
The Anatomy of Hair and Its Follicles

1. Sperling, L.C. "Hair anatomy for the clinician." *Journal of the American Academy of Dermatology* 25:(1):1–17, July 1991.

2. Montagna, W. and Ellis, R.A. (eds.) *The Biology of Hair Growth* (New York: Academic Press, 1958), p.1.

3. Fleming, R. and Mayer, T. *The Everyman's Guide to Hair Replacement* (Austin, Texas: EquiMedia Corporation, 1994), pp. 13 & 14.

4. Barman, J.M. et al. "The first stage in the natural history of the human scalp hair cycle." *Journal of Investigative Dermatology* 48:138, 1967.

5. Kligman, A.M. "Pathologic dynamics of human hair loss." *Archives of Dermatology* 83:175, 1961.

6. Saadat, M. et al. "Measurement of hair in normal newborns." *Pediatrics* 57:960, 1976.

7. Pecoraro, V. et al. "The normal trichogram in the child before puberty." *Journal of Investigative Dermatology* 42:427, 1964.

8. Gavenas, M.L. "Are you losing it?" *Glamour* August 1993, p.69.

9. Bertolino, Arthur P.; Klein, Lynn M.; and Freedberg, Irwin M. Chapter 19, "Biology of hair follicles." In *Dermatology in General Medicine,* Volume I, Fitzpatrick, Thomas B.; Eisen, Arthur Z.; Wolff, Klaus; Freedberg, Irwin M.; and Austen, K. Frank (eds), pp. 289–293.

10. Montagna, W. and Parakkal, P.F. *The Structure and Function of the Skin,* 3rd ed. (New York: Academic Press, 1974), pp. 172–258.

11. Headington, J.T. and Novak, E. "Clinical and histologic studies of male pattern baldness treated with topical minoxidil." *Current Therapeutic Research* 36:1098–1106, 1984.

12. Ebling, F.J.G. "The biology of hair." *Dermatology Clinics* 5:407–481, 1987.

13. Moschella, S.L. & Hurley, H.J. *Dermatology,* 2nd ed. (Philadelphia: W.B. Saunders, 1985), p. 1542.

14. Walker, Morton. "Clinical program to reverse male pattern baldness." *Townsend Letter for Doctors* # 83, June 1990, pp. 366–370.

15. Rabbiosi, G.; Giannetti, A.; Serri, F. "Sialic acid on the scalp of man." In Montagna, W. and Dobson, R.L.

(eds.): *Hair Growth* (London: Pergamon Press, 1969), pp. 161–168.

16. Kreysel, H.W. and Nissun, H.P. "Glycosamino glycan metabolism." In Orfanos, C.E. and Happle, R. (eds.): *Hair and Hair Diseases* (New York: Springer-Verlag, 1990), pp. 255–265.

17. Hamilton, J.B., (ed.) "The growth, replacement, and types of hair." *Annals of the New York Academy of Sciences.* vol. 53 (New York, 1951).

18. Savill, Agness Forbes. *The Hair and the Scalp.* (London, 1937).

19. *Op. cit.,* note 13, Moschella, S.L. & Hurley, H.J., p. 49.

20. Nacht, S. "Sunscreen and hair." In Lowe, N.J. (ed). *Physician's Guide to Sunscreens.* (New York: Marcel Dekker, 1991), pp 123–136.

21. Corbett, J. "Coloring and bleaching." Paper presented at the International Conference on Skin Therapy and Cosmetics, Cannes, France, 1985.

22. *Op cit.,* note 20, Nacht, S. p.130.

23. Kligman, A.M. "The human hair cycles." *J. Invest. Dermatol.* 33:307, 1959.

Chapter Four
Growth Stages of Hair and Their Problems

1. Pinkus, H. "Embrylogy of hair," in *The Biology of Hair Growth,* edited by W. Montagna and R.A. Ellis. (New York: Academic Press, 1958), p.1.

2. Montagna, W. and Parakkal, P.F. *The Structure and Function of the Skin,* 3d ed. (New York: Academic Press, 1974), pp. 172–258.

3. *Ibid.* Montagna, W. and Parakkal, P.F., p. 201.

4. Ebling, F.J.G. "The biology of hair." *Dermatol. Clin.* 5:407–481, 1987.

5. *Op cit.,* note 2, Montagna, W. and Parakkal, P.F., pp. 172–258.

6. Headington, J.T. and Novak, E. "Clinical and histologic studies of male pattern baldness treated with topical

minoxidil." *Current Therapeutic Research* 36:1098–1106, 1984.

7. Uno, H. "The histopathology of hair loss." Internet, Aug. 11, 1997, from http://npntserver.mcg.edu/html/alopecia/documents/histopathhloss.html.

8. Orentreich, N. "Scalp hair replacement in man." In Montagna, W. and Dobson, R.L. (eds) *Advances in Biology of the Skin,* vol. 9. (London: Oxford Pergamon Press, 1967), pp. 99–108.

9. Van Scott, E.J. "Keratinization and hair growth." *Annual Review of Medicine* 19:337–350, 1968.

10. Moschella, S.L. & Hurley, H.J. *Dermatology,* 3rd ed. (Philadelphia: W.B. Saunders, 1992), p. 1543.

11. Elston, D.M. and Bergfeld, W.F. "Cicatricial alopecia and other causes of permanent alopecia." In *Disorders of Hair Growth: Diagnosis and Treatment.* E.A. Olsen (ed) (New York: McGraw-Hill, Inc., 1994), p. 289.

12. *Op. cit.,* note 4, Ebling, F.J.G. pp. 407–481.

Chapter Five
Why Some Women Lose Their Hair
or See It Grow Thin

1. Suriannello, Elline. "A woman today: I'm not ashamed anymore." *Ladies Home Journal,* February 1992, p. 26.

2. Jacobs, S. *The Big Fall.* (Burnaby, BC Canada: New Century Books, 1992), p. 55.

3. Bertolino, A.P. and Freedberg, I.M. "Disorders of epidermal appendages and related disorders." In *Dermatology in General Medicine,* Volume 1, Fitzpatrick, T.B.; Eisen, A.Z.; Wolff, K.; Freedberg, I.M.; Austen, K.F. (eds). (New York: McGraw-Hill, Inc., Fourth Ed., 1993), pp. 671–695.

4. Hamilton, J.B. "Patterned long hair in man: Types and incidence." *Annals of the New York Academy of Science* 53:708, 1951.

5. Ludwig, E. "Classification of the types of androgenetic alopecia (common baldness) arising in the female sex." *British Journal of Dermatology* 97:249, 1977.

6. Lynfield, Y.L. "Effect of pregnancy on the human

hair cycle." *Journal of Investigational Dermatology* 35:323–327, 1960.

7. Randall, V.A.; Thornton, M.J.; Hamada, K.; Messenger, A.G. "Mechanism of androgen action in cultured dermal papilla cells derived from human hair follicles with varying responses to androgens *in vivo.*" *Journal of Invest. Dermatol.* 98:86S–91S, 1992.

8. King, R.J.B. "Structure and function of steroid receptors." *Journal of Endocrinol.* 114:341-349, 1987.

9. Eil, C. and Edelson, S.K. "The use of human skin fibroblasts to obtain potency estimates of drug binding to androgen receptors." *J. Clin. Endocrinol. Metab.* 59:51–55, 1984.

10. Parkinson, Richard W. "Hair loss in women." *Postgraduate Medicine* 9 (4): 417–431, March 1992.

Chapter Six
Chemotherapy as a Cause of Hair Loss

1. Schnare, D.W., et al. "Body burden reductions of PCBs, PBBs and chlorinated pesticides in human subjects." *Ambio: A Journal of the Human Environment* 13(5–6):378–380, 1984.

2. Kellas, W.R. and Dworkin, A.S. *Surviving the Toxic Crisis: Understanding, Preventing and Treating the Root Causes of Chronic Illness.* (Olivenhain, California: Professional Preference, 1996), p. 26.

3. Seipp, C.A. "Adverse effects of treatment." In *Cancer, Principles and Practice.* DeVita, V.T., Jr.; Hellman, S.; Rosenberg, S.A. (eds) (Philadelphia: J.B. Lippincott Co., 2nd Ed., 1985), pp. 2007–2008.

4. Hood, A.F. "Cutaneous side effects of cancer chemotherapy." *Med. Clin. North Am.* 70:499–503, 1986.

5. Hussein, Atif M. "Chemotherapy-induced alopecia: new developments." *Southern Medical Journal* 86 (5):489–495, May 1993.

6. Kerker, B.J. and Hood, A. F. "Chemothrapy-induced cutaneous reactions." *Seminar Dermatology* 8:173–181, 1989.

7. Bronner, A.K. and Hood, A.F. "Cutaneous complications of chemotherapeutic agents." *Journal of the American Academy of Dermatology* 9:645–663, 1983.

8. Cleveland, C.B.; Francke, D.E.; Heller, W.M., et al (eds). *AHFS Drug Information* (Bethesda, MD: American Society of Hospital Pharmacists, 1992), p. 497

9. Crounse, R.G. and Van Scott, E.J. "Changes in scalp hair roots as a measure of toxicity from cancer chemotherapeutic drugs." *Journal of Investigative Dermatology* 35:83–90, 1960.

10. *Op. cit.,* note 7, cit. Bronner, A.K. and Hood, A.F., 1983.

11. *Op. cit.,* note 6, Kerker, B.J. and Hood, A.F., 1989.

12. *Physicians' Desk Reference,* 47th ed. (Montvale, NJ: Medical Economics Data, 1993).

13. *Op. cit.,* note 7, Bronner, A.K. and Hood, A.F., 1983.

14. *Ibid.*

15. *Op. cit.,* note 9, Crounse, R.G. and Van Scott, E.J., 1960.

16. *Op. cit.,* note 6, Kerker, B.J. and Hood, A.F.,1989.

17. Falkson, G. and Schulz, E.J. "Changes in hair pigmentation associated with cancer chemotherapy." *Cancer Treatment Representative* 65:529, 1981.

18. *Op. cit.,* note 6, Kerker, B.J. and Hood, A.F., 1989.

19. Dorr. R.T. and Fritz, W.L. (eds). *Cancer Chemotherapy Handbook* (New York: Elsevier Science Publishing, 1980).

20. *Op. cit.,* note 6, Kerker, B.J. and Hood, A.F., 1989.

21. *Op. cit.,* note 12, *Physicians' Desk Reference.*

22. *Op. cit.,* note 19, Dorr, R.T. and Fritz, W.L., 1980.

23. *Ibid.*

24. Hood, A.F. "Cutaneous side effects of cancer chemotherapy." *Medical Clinics of North America* 70:187–209, 1986.

25. *Op. cit.,* note 12, *Physicians' Desk Reference.*

26. *Ibid.*

27. *Ibid.*

28. Sullivan, R.D.; Mescon, H.; Jones, R. "The effect

of intra-arterial nutrogen-mustard therapy on human skin."
Cancer 6:288–293, 1953.

29. *Op. cit.,* note 12, *Physicians' Desk Reference.*

30. *Op. cit.,* note 7, Bronner, A.K. and Hood, A.F., 1983.

31. *Op. cit.,* note 24, Hood, A.F., 1986.

32. *Op. cit.,* note 12, *Physicians' Desk Reference.*

33. *Op. cit.,* note 6, Kerker, B.J. and Hood, A.F., 1989.

34. *Op. cit.,* note 12, *Physicians' Desk Reference.*

35. *Op. cit.,* note 9, Crounse, R.G. and Van Scott, E.J., 1960.

36. *Op. cit.,* note 24, Hood, A.F., 1986.

37. *Ibid.*

38. *Op. cit.,* note 7, Bronner, A.K. and Hood, A.F., 1983.

39. Chabner, B.K. and Myers, C.E. "Clinical pharmacology of cancer chemotherapy." In *Cancer, Principles and Practice.* DeVita, V.T., Jr.; Hellman, S; Rosenberg, S.A. (eds). (Philadelphia: J.B. Lippincott Co., 2nd ed., 1985), pp. 2287–328.

40. Hubbard, S.M. "Chemotherapy-induced alopecia." *Clin. Oncology.* 4:387–457, 1985.

41. Levantine, A. and Almeyda, J. "Drug-induced alopecia." *Br. J. Dermatol.* 89:549–553, 1973.

42. Ebling, F.J.G. "The biology of hair." *Dermatol. Clin.* 5:467-481, 1987.

43. Welch, D. and Lewis, K. "Alopecia and chemotherapy." *Am. J. Nurs.* 80:903–905, 1980.

44. *Op. cit.,* note 24, Hood, A.F. 1986.

45. Chen, H.S.G. and Gross, J.F. "Physiologically based pharmacokinetics models for anticancer drugs." *Cancer Chemother. Pharmacol.* 2:85–94, 1979.

46. Falkson, G. and Schulz, E.J. "Changes in hair pigmentation associated with cancer chemotherapy." *Cancer Treat. Rep.* 65:529, 1981.

47. Witman, G.; Cadman, E.; Chen, M. "Misuse of scalp hypothermia." *Cancer Treat. Rep.* 65:507–508, 1981.

48. Simister, J.M. "Alopecia and cytotoxic drugs" *Br. Med. J.* 2:1138, 1966.

49. Hennessey, J.D. "Alopecia and cytotoxic drugs (Letter)." *British Med. J.* 1:1138, 1966.

50. Martin-Jimenez M.; Diaz-Rubio, E.; Gonzalez-Larriba, J.E., et al. "Failure of high dose tocopherol to prevent alopecia induced by doxorubicin." *N. Engl. J. Med.* 315:894–895, 1986.

51. Perez, J.E.; Macchiavelli, M.; Leone, B.A., et al. "High-dose alpha-tocopherol as a preventive of doxorubicin-induced alopecia." *Cancer Treat. Rep.* 70:1213–1214, 1986.

52. *Op. cit.,* note 9, Crounse, R.G. and Van Scott, E.J., 1960.

53. *Ibid.*

54. Sims, R.T. " 'Beau's lines' in hair: Reduction of hair shaft diameter associated with illness." *British Journal of Dermatology* 79:43–49, 1967.

55. *Op. cit.,* note 9, Crounse, R.G. and Van Scott, E.J., 1960.

56. *Op. cit.,* note 6, Kerker, B.J. and Hood, A.F., 1989.

57. Wheeland, R.G.; Burgdorf, W.H.C.; Humphrey, G.B. "The flag sign of chemotherapy." *Cancer* 51:1356–1358, 1963.

58. *Ibid.*

59. *Ibid.*

Chapter Seven
How to Stop Baldness from Cytotoxic Chemicals

1. Legwold, Gary. "Gone today, hair tomorrow: the bald facts on hair loss." *Better Homes and Gardens* March 1993, pp. 62–65.

2. U.S. Department of Health and Human Services, *Cancer Rates and Risks,* 1985.

3. American Cancer Society, *Cancer Facts and Figures,* 1991.

4. Moss, R.W. *The Cancer Industry: Unraveling the Politics* (New York: Paragon House, 1989).

5. "Progress against cancer?" *New England Journal of Medicine* May 8, 1986.

6. Morra, M. and Potts, E. *Choices: Realistic Alternatives in Cancer Treatment* (New York: Avon Books, 1980), pp.179 & 180.

7. Kellas, W.R. and Dworkin, A.S. *Thriving in a Toxic World* (Olivenhain, California: Professional Preference, 1996), p. 132.

8. Luepke, Neals Peter. "Summary report concerning adjuvant local application of *Thymu-Skin®* preparations in patients undergoing cytostatic chemotherapy." *German Journal of Oncology* 22:13–20, 1990.

9. *Ibid.*

10. Baxley, K.O.; Erdman, L.K.; Henry, E.B., et al. "Alopecia: effect on cancer patients' body image." *Cancer Nurs.* 7:499–503, 1984.

11. Wagner, L. and Bye, M.G. "Body image and patients experiencing alopecia as a result of cancer chemotherapy." *Cancer Nurs.* 2:365–369, 1979.

12. Clement-Jones, V. "Cancer and beyond: the formation of BACUP." *British Med. J.* 291:1021–1023, 1985.

Chapter Eight
Present Alopecia Treatments for Men and Women

1. *The AMA Book of Skin and Hair Care,* Schoen, L.A. ed. (Philadelphia: J.B. Lippincott Co., 1976), p. 171.

2. Segell, M. "The bald truth about hair." *Esquire* 121(5):111, May 1994.

3. *Ibid.*

4. Legwold, G., "Gone today, hair tomorrow: the bald facts on hair loss." *Better Homes and Gardens* March 1993, p. 64.

5. Fiedler-Weiss, V.C.; Rumsfield, J.; Buys, C.M.; West, D.P.; Wendrow, A. "Evaluation of oral minoxidil in the treatment of alopecia areata." *Archives of Dermatology* 123:1488–1490, 1987.

6. White, S.I. and Friedmann, P.S. "Topical minoxidil lacks efficacy in alopecia areata." [Letter]. *Archives of Dermatology* 121:591, 1985.

7. Fiedler-Weis, V.C. "Topical minoxidil solution (1% and 5%) in the treatment of alopecia areata." *Journal of the*

American Academy of Dermatology 16(Part 2 of 3):745–748, 1987.

8. Fainstein, V.; Andres, N.; Umphrey, J.; Hopfer, R. "Hair clipping: Another hazard for granulocytopenic patients?" *Journal of Infectious Diseases* 158(3):655–656, 1988.

9. O'Donoghue, M.N. "Hair cosmetics." *Dermatological Clinics* 5(3):619–626, 1987.

Chapter Nine
Using Dietary Supplements to Prevent Hair Loss

1. Thomson, B. "Man to Man: The truth about hair loss." *Natural Health* May-June 1997, p. 36.

2. Hofstein, R. and Batson, S. *Grow Hair in 12 Weeks— the Natural, Healthy Way to Save What You Have and Restore What You Don't in Less than 1 Hour a Week* (New York: Crown Publishers, Inc., 1988), p. 14–16.

3. Alexander, D. *Healthy Hair and Common Sense* (West Hartford, Connecticut: The Witkower Press, 1976), p. 66.

4. Balch, J.F. and Balch, P.A. *Prescription for Nutritional Healing,* 2nd edition (Garden City Park, NY: Avery Publishing Group, 1997), p. 16.

5. *Ibid.*

6. Lieberman, S. and Bruning, N. *The Real Vitamin & Mineral Book,* Second Edition (Garden City Park, NY: Avery Publishing Group, 1997).

7. Mindell, E. *Earl Mindell's New and Revised Vitamin Bible* (New York: Warner Books, 1985), 48–52.

8. Walker, M. "Adaptogens: Nature's answer to stress." *Townsend Letter for Doctors,* Medical Journalist Report of Innovative Biologics (monthly column), pp. 751–755, July 1994.

9. Peters, K.; Stuss, D.; Waddell, N. *Hair Loss Prevention Through Natural Remedies: A Prescription for Healthier Hair* (Vancouver, B.C.: Apple Publishing Co., Ltd., 1996), pp. 35–37.

10. *Ibid.,* pp. 47 & 48.

11. *Op. cit.,* note 8. Walker, M.

12. Brekhman, I.I. and Dardymov, I.V. "New substances of plant origin which increase nonspeific resistance." *Annual Review of Pharmacology,* Volume 9, 1969.

13. Walker, M. "Neutralizing stress and increasing stamina." *Explore!* Volume 5(5–6): 9–13, November 1994.

14. Brekhman, I.I. *Eleutherococcus.* (Leningrad: Nauka Publishing, 1968).

15. Crayhon, R. *Nutrition Made Simple* (New York: M. Evans and Company, Inc., 1996), pp. 167 & 168.

16. Balch. J.F. and Balch, P.A. *Prescription for Nutritional Healing,* Second Edition (Garden City Park, NY: Avery Publishing Group, 1997), pp. 54 & 55.

17. Scaglione, F. et al. "Immunomodulatory effects of two extracts of Panax ginseng." in *Drugs in Experimental Clinical Research* 16(10):537–542, 1990.

18. Kenarova, B. et al. "Immunomodulating activity of ginsenoside Rg1 from *Panax ginseng.*" *Japanese Journal of Pharmacology* 54(4):447–454, 1990.

19. Jie, Y.H.; Cammisuli, S.; Baggiolini, M. "Immunomodulatory effects of *Panax ginseng* in the mouse." *Agents Actions* 15(3–4):386–391, 1984.

20. Bohn, B.; Nebe, C.T.; Birr, C. "Flow-cytometric studies with *Eleutherococcus senticosus* extract as an immunomodulatory agent." *Arzneim-Forsch* 37(10):1193–1196, 1987.

Chapter Ten
The Ultimate Nutritional Drink
to Stop Falling Hair

1. Walker, M. "The soybean concentrate from China for reversing metastatic cancer." *Explore! for the Professional* 7(2):29–33, December 1996.

2. Walker, M. "Chinese soybean concentrate, the ultimate in healing foods." *Healthy & Natural Journal* 3(3):68–69, June 1996.

3. Walker, M. "Haelan 851® as anticancer nutrition." *Explore More!* 14:5–8, Sept. 1996.

4. Walker, M. "Therapeutics of soybean extract." *Explore! for the Professional* 6(3):40–43, June 1995.

5. Walker, M. "Concentrated soybean phytochemicals." *Healthy & Natural Journal,* 2(2):58–60, April 1995.

6. Walker, M. "Phytochemicals in soybeans" (*Nutritional Medicine* monthly column) *Health Foods Business,* March 1995, p. 36.

7. Walker, M. "Soybean isoflavones lower risks of degenerative diseases." *(Medical Journalist Report of Innovative Biologics* monthly column) *Townsend Letter for Doctors,* August/September 1994, pp. 874–878.

8. Mitchell, A.J. and Krull, E.A. "Alopecia areata: Pathogenesis and treatment." *Journal of the American Academy of Dermatology* 11:763–775, 1984.

9. Hordinsky, M.A. "Alopecia areata" In Jordan, R.E. (ed): *Immunologic Diseases of the Skin.* (East Norwalk, CT: Appleton and Lange, 1991), pp. 427–434.

10. Nelson, D.A. and Spielvogel, R.L. "Alopecia areata" (review). *International Journal of Dermatology* 24:26–34, 1985.

11. Aw, T.C. and Cheah, J.S. "Diabetes mellitus presenting with alopecia areata totalis (letter)." *Lancet* 1(2):268, 1978.

12. Schonwetter, R.S. and Nelson,E.B. "Alopecia areata and the acquired-immunodeficiency-syndrome-related-complex." *Annuals of Internal Medicine* 104:287, 1986.

13. Ostlere, L.S.; Langry, J.A.A.; Staughton, R.C.D.; Samrasinghe, P.L. "Alopecia universalis in a patient seropositive for the human immunodeficiency virus." *Journal of the American Academy of Dermatology* 27:630–631, 1992.

14. Brown, A.C.; Pollard, Z.F.; Jarrett, W.H. "Ocular and testicular abnormalities in alopecia areata." *Archives of Dermatology* 118:546–554, 1982.

15. Koshland, D.E. "Recognizing self from nonself." *Science* 248:1273, 1990.

16. Stine, G.J. *Acquired Immune Deficiency Syndrome* (Englewood Cliffs, NJ: Prentice Hall, 1993), p. 12.

17. Headington, J.T. "The histopathology of alopecia

areata (abstract)." *Journal of Investigative Dermatology* 96:69S, 1991.

18. MacDonald-Hull, S.P., et al. "Immunohistologic and ultrastructural comparison of the dermal papilla and hair follicle bulb from 'active' and 'normal' areas of alopecia areata." *Journal of Investigative Dermatology* 96:673–681, 1991.

19. Tobin, D.J.; Fenton, D.A.; Kendall, M.D. "Cell degeneration in alopecia areata." *American Journal of Dermatopathology* 13:248–256, 1991.

20. Brocker, E-B; Echternacht-Happle, K.; Hamm, H.; Happle, R. "Abnormal expression of class I and class II major histocompatibility antigens in alopecia areata: Modulation by topical immunotherapy." *Journal of Investigative Dermatology* 88:564–568, 1987.

21. Khoury, E.L.; Price, VH.; Greenspan, J.S. "HLA-DR expression by hair follicle keratinocytes in alopecia areata: Evidence that it is secondary to the lymphoid infiltration." *Journal of Investigative Dermatology* 90:193–200, 1988.

22. Nickoloff, B.J. and Griffiths, C.E.M. "Aberrant intercellular adhesion molecule-1 (ICAM-1) expression by hair follicle epithelial cells and endothelial leukocyte adhesion molecule-1 (ELAM-1) by vascular cells are important adhesion-molecule alterations in alopecia areata." *Journal of Investigational Dermatology* 96:91S–92S, 1991.

23. Dustin, L.M.; Singer, K.H.; Tuck, D.T.; Springer, T.A. "Adhesion of T-lymphoblasts to epidermal keratinocytes is regulated by interferon gamma and is mediated by intercellular adhesion molecule (ICAM-1)." *Experimental Medicine* 167:1323–1340, 1988.

24. *Op. cit.,* note 1. Walker, M. "The soybean concentrate from China for reversing metastatic cancer." *Explore! for the Professional* 7(2):29–33, December 1996.

25. Okubo, K.; Kudou, S.; Uchida, T.; Yoshiki, Y.; Yoshikoshi, M.; Tonomura, M. "Soybean saponin and isoflavonoid: Structure and antiviral activity against human immunodeficiency virus in vitro." In *Food Phytochemicals for Cancer Prevention, Volume I, Fruits and Vegetables.* Huang, M-T.; Osawa, T.; HO, C-Tan.; Rosen, R.T. (eds.)

(Washington, D.C.: American Chemical Society, 1994), pp. 330–339.

26. Kurihara, M.; Aoki, K.; Hisamichi, F. *UICC Publication* (Nagoya, Japan: Nagoya University Press, 1989).

27. Nair, P.N.; Turjuman, N.; Kessie, G.; Calkins, B.; Goodman, G.T.; Davitvitz, H.; Nimmagadda, G. *Am. J. Clin. Nutr.* 40:927–930, 1984.

28. Messina, Mark and Barnes, Stephen. *Journal of the National Cancer Institute* 83:541–546, 1991.

Chapter Eleven
General Therapeutic Effects of
Calf Thymus Extract

1. Weiner, M.A. and Goss, K. *Maximum Immunity* (Boston: Houghton Mifflin Co., 1986), p. 214.

2. Tobin, D.J.; Orentreich, N.; Fenton, D.A.; Bystryn, J-C. "Antibodies to hair follicles in alopecia areata." *The Journal of Investigative Dermatology* 102(5):721–724, May 1994.

3. Brystryn, J-CI and Tamesis, J. "Immunologic aspects of hair loss." *Journal of Investigative Dermatology* 96:88S–89S, 1991.

4. Sato, S. "Ultrastructural study of alopecia areata." In: Toda, K.; Ishibashi, Y.; Hori, Y.; Morikawa, F. (eds.). *Biology and Disease of the Hair.* (Tokyo: University of Tokyo Press, 1976), pp. 295–304.

5. Kohchiyama, A.; Hatamochi, A.; Ueki, H. "Increased numbers of OKT-6-postive dendritic cells in the hair follicles of patients with alopecia areata." *Dermatologica* 171:327–331, 1985.

6. Bystryn, J-C; Orentreich, N.; Stengel, F. "Direct immunofluorescence studies in alopecia areata and male pattern alopecia." *Journal of Investigational Dermatology* 73:317–320, 1979.

7. Khoury, E.L.; Price, V.H.; Greenspan, J.S. "HLA-DR expression by hair follicle keratinocytes in alopecia areata: Evidence that it is secondary to the lymphoid infiltration." *Journal of Investigational Dermatology* 90:193–200, 1988.

8. *Op. cit.*, note 3, Brystryn, J-C and Tamesis, J., 1991.

9. Helm, F. and Milgrom, H. "Can scalp hair suddenly turn white? A case of canities subita." *Archives of Dermatology* 102:102–103, 1970.

10. Messenger, A.G. and Bleehan, S.S. "Alopecia areata: Light and electron microscopic pathology of the regrowing white hair." *British Journal of Dermatology* 110:155–162, 1984.

11. Tosti, A.; Columbati, S.; Caponeeri, G.M.; Ciliberti, C.; Tosti, G.; Bosi, M.; Veronesi, S. "Ocular abnormalities occurring with alopecia areata." *Dermatologica* 170:69–73, 1985.

12. White, A. "The endocrine role of the thymus and its hormone thymosin, in immunological competence," presented at the National Foundation March of Dimes, Harbor Springs, Michigan, USA, 1975.

13. Goldstein, A. "Preparation of active thymosin," *Proc. Natl. Acad. Science* 69:1800, 1972.

14. Goldstein, S. "Biological aging: an essentially normal process." *J.A.M.A.* 195:30, 1974.

15. Cooper, J.A. "Extraction of active thymosin from calf thymus." *Ann NY Acad. Science* 1976.

16. Czaplicki, J.; Blonska, B.; Czarnecki, J.; Pesic, M.C. "Do active substances of the thymus influence the processes of aging? Effect of prothymosis alpha-1 and mature thymic extracts (TFX and thymex-L) on the amount of purkinje cells in old mice cerebellum." *International Journal of Thymology* 1(2):83–93, October 1993.

17. Inderst, R. "Experience with combinations of thymus extract and enzymes in the treatment of autoimmune diseases, viral infections and tumours." *International J. Thymology* 2(3):142–148, April 1994.

Chapter Twelve
Studies on Thymus Extract to Reverse Alopecia

1. Moessler, K. "Thymu-Skin: Neuer Therapieansatz bei der Behandlung der Alopecia androgenetica und der Alopecia areata." *Deutsche Dermat.* 39:945–956, 1991.

2. Moessler, K. ''Behandlung der Alopecia androgenetica und der Alopecia areata mit thymusextrakthaltigen External.'' *Erfahrungsheilkunde* 3:144–149, 1993.

3. Moessler, K. and Hagedorn, M. ''Local therapy with thymus extract in patients with alopecia areata totalis and universalis.'' *German Dermat.*, pp. 3–8, 1993.

4. *Ibid.* Moessler and Hagedorn, p. 7.

5. Fleming, R.W. and Mayer, T.G. *The Everyman's Guide to Hair Replacement* (Austin, Texas: EquiMedia Corp., 1994), p. 26.

6. *Ibid.*, p. 25.

7. Dauber, R. and Van Neste, D. *Hair and Scalp Disorders: Common Presenting Signs, Differential Diagnosis and Treatment* (Philadelphia: J.B. Lippincott Company, 1995), pp. 169–170.

8. *Op. cit.*, note 5, Fleming, R. and Mayer, T., pp.15–16

Chapter Thirteen
The Hair-Preserving Properties of *Thymu-Skin*®

1. Pullmann, H., ''Thymusextrakte bei verschiedenen Formen der Alopezie.'' Dermatologie Heute (Berlin) Mai 1992, p. 1.

2. ''Salz, Sonne und Wind schaden dem Haar im Urlaub braucht es besondere Pflege.'' *Das Neue Blatt* Nr. 26, 20 Juni 1990, p. 12.

3. Sadick, N.S. and Richardson, D.C. *Your Hair: Helping to Keep It.* (New York: Consumer Reports Books, 1991), pp. 46–47.

ABOUT THE AUTHOR

MORTON WALKER, D.P.M. A doctor of podiatric medicine, Dr. Morton Walker now writes full-time as a professional freelance medical journalist. He has published seventy-one books (including fourteen 100,000-copy bestsellers) and nearly 2,000 consumer magazine, clinical journal, and newspaper articles. Each month, he writes columns for five medically oriented periodicals: two American holistic clinical journals, two consumer health magazines, and a trade journal of the health foods industry. His books are published in twenty-eight countries, and the number continues to grow.

Dr. Walker has been featured by, or appeared as a guest with, Regis Philbin and Kathie Lee Gifford, Oprah Winfrey, Mike Douglas, Merv Griffin, Sally Jesse Raphael, Jay Leno, and other television talk show hosts. Dr. Walker specializes in those health care sciences referred to as orthomolecular nutrition, holistic (biological) medicine, and alternative methods of healing.

The winner of twenty-three (23) medical journalism awards and medals, Dr. Walker was recognized with the 1992 *Humanitarian Award* from the American Cancer Control Society, which named him: "The world's leading medical journalist specializing in holistic medicine."

He received the 1981 *Orthomolecular Award* from the American Institute of Preventive Medicine, for his "outstanding achievement in orthomolecular education."

He was presented with the 1979 *Humanitarian Award* from the 1,100 physician-members of the American College for Advancement in Medicine "for informing the American public on alternative methods of healing."

He has received two prestigious Jesse H. Neal *Editorial Achievement Awards* from the American Business Press, Inc., for creating the best series of magazine articles published in any audited United States magazine in both 1975 and 1976.

HEALTH CARE BOOKS FROM KENSINGTON

EAT HEALTHY WITH KENSINGTON

COOKING WITHOUT RECIPES
by Cheryl Sindell   (1-57566-142-X, $13.00/$18.00)
Unleash your creativity and prepare meals your friends and family
will love with the help of this innovative kitchen companion. COOK-
ING WITHOUT RECIPES includes intriguing culinary strategies and
nutritional secrets that will stir your imagination and put the fun back
into cooking.

DINING IN THE RAW   (1-57566-192-6, $19.95/$24.95)
by Rita Romano
The first recipe book that explores high-enzyme living using raw
food cuisine. Complete with over 700 delicious recipes for entrees,
salads, soups, desserts, sauces and dressings, it explains how healthy
eating can actually help cure chronic ailments such as allergies, skin
disorders, arthritis, mood swings, colds, digestive problems and more
. . . *without* counting every calorie!

EAT HEALTHY FOR $50 A WEEK
Feed Your Family Nutritious, Delicious Meals for Less
by Rhonda Barfield   (1-57566-018-0, $12.00/$15.00)
Filled with dozens of recipes, helpful hints, and sample shopping
lists, EAT HEALTHY FOR $50 A WEEK is an indispensable hand-
book for balancing your budget and stretching your groceries while
feeding your family healthy and nutritious meals.

THE ARTHRITIC'S COOKBOOK
by Collin H. Dong, M.D.   (1-57566-158-6, $9.95/$12.95)
and Jane Banks
Afflicted with debilitating, "incurable" arthritis, Dr. Collin H. Dong
decided to fight back. Combining traditional Chinese folk wisdom
with his western medical practice, he created a diet that made his
painful symptoms disappear. Today, used in conjunction with regular
arthritis medications, this groundbreaking diet has provided thousands
of Dr. Dong's patients with active, happy, and virtually pain-free lives.
It can do the same for you.

*Available wherever paperbacks are sold, or order direct from the
Publisher. Send cover price plus 50¢ per copy for mailing and
handling to Kensington Publishing Corp., Consumer Orders,
or call (toll free) 888-345-BOOK, to place your order using
Mastercard or Visa. Residents of New York and Tennessee
must include sales tax. DO NOT SEND CASH.*